DATE DUE

Nutrition and Obesity

Assessment, Management & Prevention

Alexandra G. Kazaks, PhD, RD

Assistant Professor
Department of Nutrition and Exercise Science
Bastyr University

Judith S. Stern, RD, ScD

Distinguished Professor
Departments of Nutrition and Internal Medicine
University of California at Davis

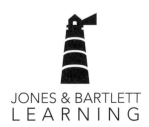

JONES & BARTLETT
LEARNING

World Headquarters
Jones & Bartlett Learning
5 Wall Street
Burlington, MA 01803
978-443-5000
info@jblearning.com
www.jblearning.com

Jones & Bartlett Learning books and products are available through most bookstores and online booksellers. To contact Jones & Bartlett Learning directly, call 800-832-0034, fax 978-443-8000, or visit our website, www.jblearning.com.

Nutrition and Obesity: Assessment, Management, and Prevention is an independent publication and has not been authorized, sponsored, or otherwise approved by the owners of the trademarks or service marks referenced in this product.

Some images in this book feature models. These models do not necessarily endorse, represent, or participate in the activities represented in the images.

The authors, editor, and publisher have made every effort to provide accurate information. However, they are not responsible for errors, omissions, or for any outcomes related to the use of the contents of this book and take no responsibility for the use of the products and procedures described. Treatments and side effects described in this book may not be applicable to all people; likewise, some people may require a dose or experience a side effect that is not described herein. Drugs and medical devices are discussed that may have limited availability controlled by the Food and Drug Administration (FDA) for use only in a research study or clinical trial. Research, clinical practice, and government regulations often change the accepted standard in this field. When consideration is being given to use of any drug in the clinical setting, the health care provider or reader is responsible for determining FDA status of the drug, reading the package insert, and reviewing prescribing information for the most up-to-date recommendations on dose, precautions, and contraindications, and determining the appropriate usage for the product. This is especially important in the case of drugs that are new or seldom used.

Production Credits
Publisher: Cathleen Sether
Executive Editor: Shoshanna Goldberg
Editorial Assistant: Agnes Burt
Production Manager: Julie Champagne Bolduc
Production Editor: Joanna Lundeen
Marketing Manager: Andrea DeFronzo
VP, Manufacturing and Inventory Control: Therese Connell
Composition: Laserwords Private Limited, Chennai, India
Cover Design: Scott Moden
Associate Rights and Photo Researcher: Amy Rathburn
Printing and Binding: Edwards Brothers Malloy
Cover Printing: Edwards Brothers Malloy

Library of Congress Cataloging-in-Publication Data
Kazaks, Alexandra G.
  Nutrition and obesity: assessment, management, and prevention / Alexandra G. Kazaks, Judith S. Stern.
    p. ; cm.
  Includes bibliographical references and index.
  ISBN 978-0-7637-7850-7
  I. Stern, Judith S., 1943- II. Title.
  [DNLM: 1. Obesity. 2. Nutrition Therapy. WD 210]

  616.3'98—dc23
                                                           2012006816

Printed in the United States of America
16 15 14 13 12   10 9 8 7 6 5 4 3 2 1

CONTENTS

PREFACE

Obesity is a condition in which excess body fat may compromise health.

—NHLBI, 1998

Why is obesity such an important issue? Shouldn't the condition be resolved by adequate and appropriate knowledge, or a little more willpower? Consider these health statistics:

- Two out of three adults in the United States are overweight or obese.
- Over the past two decades the number of people in the highest categories of obesity increased dramatically.
- Obesity rates have increased in all groups regardless of age, sex, education, ethnicity, socioeconomic status, or geographic location. Since the 1980s the rate of obesity has doubled in adults and tripled in children, and it is now higher than at any other time in history (CDC, 2010).
- Permanent weight loss is unattainable for most people. Nearly 80% of dieters regain lost weight within 1 year (Wing, 2005).

In 2004, Surgeon General Richard Carmona made an astonishing statement regarding the seriousness of the increase in childhood obesity: "Because of the increasing rates of obesity, unhealthy eating habits, and physical inactivity, we may see the first generation that will be less healthy and have a shorter life expectancy than their parents." Accumulation of excess body weight at a young age has been linked to higher and earlier death rates in adulthood (Krebs, 2007). Obesity has a significant impact on health and longevity as it is linked to more than 60 chronic diseases such as diabetes, arthritis, sleep apnea, and hypertension (NHBLI, 1998). In national debates about healthcare reform, policymakers are increasingly focused on the roles that obesity, diabetes, and other chronic diseases play in driving up healthcare costs and diminishing citizen health status. Taxpayers, governments, and businesses spend an estimated $147 billion in obesity-related medical costs (Finkelstein, 2009). It is clear that the responses and responsibility of government, media, communities, and individuals must be defined and assigned in the search for a permanent solution to the issue of obesity.

Obesity is not a recent phenomenon. Its origins can be traced back to prehistoric human ancestors as archeologists have uncovered stone and ceramic artifacts that portray obese figures. In the past, obesity has been presented in art, literature, and medical opinion as both a highly desirable form of beauty and an unhealthy condition to be avoided. Hippocrates, regarded as the father of medicine, declared that fatter individuals were more susceptible to sudden death when compared to lean people. Chronicles from the Middle Ages often describe obese individuals as wealthy and powerful. Rubens, a famed seventeenth-century artist, is known for his paintings of robust women, with obvious rolls of fat, who were rendered to convey idealized feminine beauty.

The current concern about obesity is the result of our changing lifestyles. Throughout human history obtaining enough food for survival was a major challenge that required continual physical activity. Technological advances and changes in environmental and living conditions mean that food is now much more easily available. The Centers for Disease Control and Prevention (CDC) reports that many Americans live in an obesogenic environment, that is, one characterized by abundant food availability and decreased need for physical activity.

Obesity is not a consequence of any single factor. It is the result of multiple interactions among genetic tendencies, behavior, and environment. Therefore, successful management and prevention of obesity will involve a range of long-term interventions at the individual and societal levels. Strategies could include all phases of obesity treatment from weight loss, weight maintenance, and management of obesity-related health conditions as well as a major focus on primary prevention. All interventions should be part of an integrated approach that includes an overall goal of healthy eating and regular physical activity for everyone, regardless of weight.

This is an important time in the study of obesity. Current research draws investigators from the fields of genetics, physiology, behavior, politics, and economics. The results of these studies will provide a guide for new and innovative approaches for obesity prevention and treatment (Wyatt, 2006). With half of the American population overweight and one-third obese, it is essential for health professionals to become knowledgeable about new tactics for obesity management. This text explores the biological, economic, and social problems, as well as potential remedies associated with rapidly escalating levels of obesity in the United States and throughout the world.

Section 1, Chapters 1 through 4, provides the background for assessing and understanding the determinants of obesity in adults and children in the United States and throughout the world.

General objectives include:

- Review U.S. obesity trends in current and historical context.
- Describe where to find information about obesity trends.
- Discuss associations between sex, ethnicity, socioeconomic status, and occurrence of obesity.
- Evaluate types of assessment of weight status and body composition, including appropriate methodologies and reference data for adults and children.
- Compare key theories related to the etiology of overweight and obesity, including the biologic and genetic determinants of obesity.
- Explain how current environmental factors contribute to the increase in obesity in the United States and around the world.
- Describe the medical, economic, and psychosocial consequences of obesity.
- Acknowledge the increased healthcare costs of obesity and obesity-related diseases.

Section 2, Chapters 5 through 11, describes current nutrition, activity, behavioral, pharmaceutical, and surgical approaches to obesity management. This section explores the benefits and limitations of obesity treatment and prevention strategies for individuals and for the entire population. Among the topics presented in this section are evaluations of diet plans, weight-loss supplements, pharmacological agents, and surgical options. Not only are the physical activity and behavioral aspects of weight management discussed, but the responsibilities that healthcare providers, individuals, families, and corporate and public health agencies have for obesity prevention are as well. The final chapter explores emerging and novel areas of obesity research that include links between obesity and intestinal bacteria, specific viruses, and environmental obesogens as well as the impact of sleep disturbances and social networks on weight management.

The textbook is meant to provide a foundation for in-depth discussion and to offer guidelines for integration of new information and research into practice. References, resources, and links are provided for support and for further study. PowerPoint Lecture Outlines and a Test Bank are available to all instructors adopting this text.

REFERENCES

Carmona R. *The Growing Epidemic of Childhood Obesity.* Subcommittee on Competition, Infrastructure and Foreign Commerce, Science, and Transportation. Washington, DC: Department of Health and Human Services; 2004.

CDC. Centers for Disease Control and Prevention. Behavioral Risk Factor Surveillance System Survey Data Trends 1976–1980 Through 2007–2008. 2010; http://www.cdc.gov/nchs/data/hestat/obesity_adult_07_08/obesity_adult_07_08.htm. Accessed August 15, 2011.

Finkelstein EA, Trogdon JG, Cohen JW, Dietz W. Annual medical spending attributable to obesity: payer- and service-specific estimates. *Health Aff (Millwood).* Sep–Oct 2009;28(5):w822–w831.

Krebs NF, Himes JH, Jacobson D, Nicklas TA, Guilday P, Styne D. Assessment of child and adolescent overweight and obesity. *Pediatrics.* Dec 2007;120 Suppl 4:S193–S228.

NHLBI. Clinical guidelines on the identification, evaluation, and treatment of overweight and obesity in adults: executive summary. Expert Panel on the Identification, Evaluation, and Treatment of Overweight in Adults. *Am J Clin Nutr.* Oct 1998;68(4):899–917.

Wing RR, Phelan S. Long-term weight loss maintenance. *Am J Clin Nutr.* Jul 2005;82(1 Suppl):222S–225S.

Wyatt SB, Winters KP, Dubbert PM. Overweight and obesity: prevalence, consequences, and causes of a growing public health problem. *Am J Med Sci.* Apr 2006;331(4):166–174.

About the Authors

ALEXANDRA G. KAZAKS

Alexandra G. Kazaks has a PhD in nutritional biology from the University of California at Davis. Dr. Kazaks is a respected nutrition consultant for national health and business organizations and frequently appears as a featured speaker, lecturing about diabetes, cardiovascular disease, and weight management. In addition to numerous research articles, she is coauthor of *Obesity: A Reference Handbook* (2009). Dr. Kazaks is currently a professor at Bastyr University.

JUDITH S. STERN

Judith S. Stern has a PhD in nutrition from the Harvard University School of Public Health. Dr. Stern, a highly respected member of her field, is a member of the prestigious Institute of Medicine of the National Academy of Sciences and a fellow of the American Association for the Advancement of Sciences. She frequently lectures about obesity and its impact on other diseases such as diabetes, heart disease, and certain cancers. Along with Dr. Kazaks, she is coauthor of *Obesity: A Reference Handbook* (2009). She has published almost 300 scientific papers and written more than 150 articles about obesity in magazines such as *Vogue* and *Prevention*. She is currently a distinguished professor emeritus at the University of California at Davis.

Acknowledgments

We would like to thank the professors and teachers who provided us with feedback as we developed this book. Their comments and suggestions were an invaluable aspect of the writing process. A warm thank you to Amy Allen-Chabot, PhD, RD; Dr. Nikhil Dhurandhar; Susan K. Okonkowski, MPH, RD, CCP; Eric Sternlicht, PhD; and Cindy L. Swann, MS, RD, CDE, for your suggestions and insights.

We would like to thank the students who have helped us develop this book. They have contributed greatly through conversations and class projects about new ideas and techniques that may help patients, clients, and the general public prevent or manage obesity.

We are appreciative of the students who have responded with enthusiasm and have challenged us to provide meaningful test questions and exercises in class and for this text.

Special thanks and recognition goes to Melanie Dorion, a talented research assistant who contributed valuable research and insight for this text.

EPIDEMIOLOGY, ASSESSMENT, CAUSES, AND RISKS ASSOCIATED WITH PRESENCE OF OVERWEIGHT AND OBESITY

CHAPTER 1

CURRENT OBESITY TRENDS

READER OBJECTIVES

- Estimate the current prevalence of overweight and obesity in the United States
- Summarize trends in obesity over the past 25 years
- Classify the epidemiology of overweight and obesity as they relate to geographic region
- Assess effects of the current increase in childhood obesity
- Investigate the epidemiology of overweight and obesity as they relate to sex, ethnicity, and socioeconomic status
- Describe global trends in overweight and obesity

CHAPTER OUTLINE

Obesity Prevalence in the United States

In 2010 an estimated two-thirds (67%) of US adults could be classified as either overweight or obese. Of those, about 34% were in the obese category (Flegal, 2010). That means that there are as many Americans who are obese as those who are just overweight. Since the 1980s, obesity rates for adults have doubled and rates for children have tripled. Prevalence of obesity has increased among all groups regardless of age, sex, ethnicity, socioeconomic status (SES), or geographic region. The United States maps in **Figure 1.1**, which can also be found on the Centers for Disease Control (CDC) website, display how obesity prevalence in the United States has changed over the past decades. The CDC website address is listed in the Resources section of this chapter. The map in **Figure 1.2** shows state-by-state rates of obesity in 2010. In that year, CDC surveys reported that adult obesity rates increased in 23 states and did not decrease

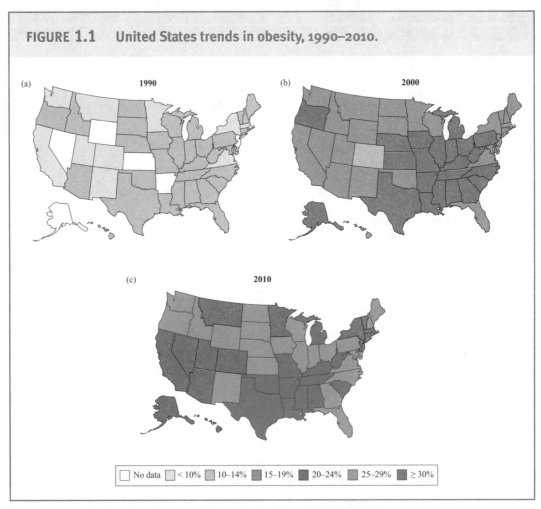

FIGURE **1.1**   United States trends in obesity, 1990–2010.

(a) 1990

(b) 2000

(c) 2010

☐ No data   ☐ < 10%   ☐ 10–14%   ☐ 15–19%   ☐ 20–24%   ☐ 25–29%   ☐ ≥ 30%

Source: Centers for Disease Control and Prevention. Obesity Trends Among U.S. Adults, BRFSS, 1990, 2000, 2010.

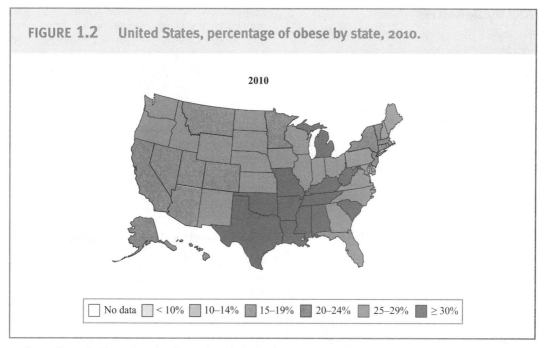

FIGURE **1.2**   United States, percentage of obese by state, 2010.

2010

No data   < 10%   10–14%   15–19%   20–24%   25–29%   ≥ 30%

Source: Centers for Disease Control and Prevention. Obesity Trends Among U.S. Adults, BRFSS, 2010.

in a single state. Obesity was most common in Mississippi where 34% of adults were obese and most uncommon in Colorado at 21%.

Animated yearly maps provided on the CDC website provide two interesting ways to examine the obesity trends data: by looking at the changes in **body mass index (BMI)** over time and at the variation in BMI among the states. In 1985, although not all states participated in the CDC survey, none that reported had an obesity rate above 15%. Compare that to 2010 when no state had a rate of obesity of less than 20% and a dozen states had a prevalence of 30% or more. The percentage of adults who were obese was more than double the percentage 25 years earlier. A striking feature of the animated maps is that they clearly show how the rate of obesity over the years appears to increase and spread with the characteristic of a communicable disease. It seems like an epidemic that is initiated in states in the Southeast. The maps' color legend draws attention to the fact that obesity continued to increase in all

states, and obesity prevalence in states with the highest rates got higher and higher over time. For details about the percentage of obesity in the individual states, view the State Obesity Rates table available on the CDC website; see the Trends by State listing in the Resources section at the end of this chapter.

One statistic not shown in these maps, but of even greater concern, is that in 30 states the percentage of obese or overweight children was 30% or more. In addition, men, women, and children of all education and income levels and from various ethnic groups were affected by the epidemic of overweight and obesity. A close look at the data showed that men and women with a college degree were less likely to be obese than those with some college education. Risk for obesity was lower in college-educated women compared with those with less than a high school diploma. To find out more about obesity trends according to economic and cultural status look at the obesity trends websites listed in the Resources section of this chapter.

Obesity Definition

For adults, overweight and obesity ranges are determined by using an individual's weight and height in an equation to calculate BMI. An adult who has a BMI between 25 and 29.9 is considered overweight. An adult who has a BMI of 30 or higher is considered obese. (That is roughly 30 or more pounds over a healthy weight.) Children are classified as overweight or obese based on where they fall on childhood BMI growth charts. Websites with more information about adult and childhood obesity assessment are listed in the Resources section of this chapter.

How Obesity Data Are Collected

Two major sources of data on the prevalence of obesity in the United States are the National Health and Nutrition Examination Survey (NHANES) and the Behavioral Risk Factor Surveillance System (BRFSS). The data from NHANES are considered the gold standard for evaluating obesity prevalence because the ongoing survey includes a household interview and a physical examination for each participant. During the physical examination, conducted in mobile examination centers, height and weight are measured along with a more a comprehensive assessment of body composition taken by trained health technicians using standardized measuring procedures and equipment. The BRFSS data comes from telephone interviews conducted each month by state health departments in all 50 states, the District of Columbia, Puerto Rico, the United States Virgin Islands, and Guam. BRFSS, established in 1984 by the CDC, is intended to be a nationally representative sample that provides state-by-state data on health issues. More than 350,000 adults are interviewed each year, making the BRFSS the largest health survey collected by telephone in the world. A drawback of the BRFSS method is that the survey data come from self-reports. Given the known inaccuracies of self-reported height and weight, the likely product of BRFSS data analysis is probably an underestimate of the actual prevalence of obesity. Self-reported weight and height compared with directly measured weight and height was evaluated in a sample from the second National Health and Nutrition Examination Survey of 1976–1980. The data showed trends of underreporting for weight and overreporting for height. Although the reported measures on average had only small errors, self-reported weight and height were more variable in key population subgroups. Misrepresentation in self-reported weight and height was directly related to a person's overweight status. Self-reported weight errors were greater in overweight females than in overweight males. As these inaccuracies in height and weight can cause significant mistakes in calculation of body mass index, direct measurement of height and weight should be performed whenever possible.

Trends in Obesity: Increasing or Leveling Off?

Between 1960 and 1980 the obesity rate was comparatively stable in the United States and about 15% of the population fell into the category. Obesity so sharply increased for the next decade that researchers were predicting that by 2020 almost half of United States adults would meet the criteria for obesity (Stewart, 2009). Then, in 2010, an analysis of NHANES data suggested that the decades-long yearly increases in overweight and obesity had slowed or perhaps had reached a plateau. Compared with the previous 10-year period, the report (Flegal, 2010) showed:

- 32.2% of men were obese, compared with 27% in 1999. However, there had been no significant change in obesity rates since 2003.
- 35.5% of women were obese compared with 33.4% in 1999. The increase was not statistically significant.
- 31.7% of children were obese or overweight compared with 29% in 1999. This increase also was not a statistically significant difference.

Even though these findings of slowed increases in overweight and obesity were good news, the statistics are still overwhelming. Most Americans are overweight and one-third of Americans are obese. Epidemiologists with the CDC's National Center for Health Statistics report that, although the obesity trend appears to be slowing down, the prevalence remains unacceptably high and obesity continues to be a serious national health concern (CDC, *Behavioral Risk*, 2010).

Extreme Obesity

The most rapid growth in obesity has occurred in the sector of the obese adult population who has **extreme or severe obesity**, with a BMI of 40 or greater and more than 100 lb of extra weight. In a study of extreme weight category trends between the years 1986 and 2000 the prevalence of a BMI of 40 or greater quadrupled from about 1 in 200 adult Americans to 1 in 50. The prevalence of a BMI of 50 or greater had a five-fold increase, from about 1 individual in 2,000 to 1 in 400. This increase included males and females, all ethnic groups, all age groups, and all education levels. Those with the highest BMI at the baseline measurement had the greatest increases. The heaviest people gained the most weight (Sturm, 2003). This effect is apparent in **Table 1.1**, Prevalence of Overweight, Obesity, and Extreme Obesity. Although a comparison of BMI categories during the period from 1960 to 2006 showed no significant increase in the prevalence of overweight, it demonstrated about a two-and-a-half-fold rise in obesity and a nearly sevenfold increase in extreme obesity.

Childhood Obesity

The prevalence of overweight and obesity in children and adolescents has increased in parallel with that in adults in the United States since 1980. The 2007–2008 NHANES data indicated that almost 32% of school-aged children and adolescents were categorized as overweight and almost 17% were obese (Ogden, 2010). The **childhood overweight** category is defined as at or above the 85th percentile of weight for age (CDC, *Basics*, 2010). The **childhood obesity** category is a BMI at or above the 95th weight percentile for a specific age. The prevalence of BMI-for-age values ≥95th percentile (obesity category) in adolescents 12 to 19 years of age was 18% in 2008 compared with 6% in the 1971–1974 NHANES. The increase was also seen in young children 6 to 11 years of age. Compared with 4% in 1971, the rate was five times more, at 20% in 2008 (Ogden, 2010). Even infants and children between 6 and 23 months old are getting heavier. The prevalence of high weight for age for this group was 7% in the 1976–1980 report and 12% in 2006 (NCHS, 2010).

Children who are overweight or obese are at increased risk of developing heart disease, type 2 diabetes, stroke, and asthma during childhood, and

TABLE 1.1	Prevalence of Overweight, Obesity, and Extreme Obesity		
	Overweight (BMI 25–29.9)	**Obese (BMI 30–39.9)**	**Extremely obese (BMI 40 or above)**
1960–1962	31.5%	13.4%	0.9%
1971–1974	32.3%	14.5%	1.3%
1976–1989	32.1%	15.0%	1.4%
1988–1994	32.7%	23.2%	3.0%
1999–2000	33.6%	30.9%	5.0%
2001–2002	34.4%	31.3%	5.4%
2003–2004	33.4%	32.9%	5.1%
2005–2006	32.2%	35.1%	6.2%

Modified from: Prevalence of overweight, obesity and extreme obesity among adults: United States, trends 1960–62 through 2005–2006. Health E-Stats, CDC, December 2008; http://www.cdc.gov/nchs/data/hestat/overweight/overweight_adult.pdf.

they are likely to become obese adults (Daniels, 2005). Overweight adolescents have a 70% chance of becoming overweight adults. The risk increases to 80% if one or both parents are overweight or obese (NCHS, 2010). While optimal levels of BMI related to long-term health in children and teens are not actually known, the prevalence of obesity in youth will most likely result in population-wide increases in obesity-associated disorders in the future. In 2010, as an update to previous warnings about childhood obesity, United States Surgeon General Regina Benjamin declared, "If we do not reverse these trends, researchers warn that many of our children—our most precious resource—will be seriously afflicted in early adult-hood with medical conditions such as diabetes and heart disease. This future is unacceptable" (Benjamin, 2010).

In 2008 some promising statistics emerged. After years of steady increases, data from the CDC showed that rates of childhood overweight did not increase between the 1999–2000 and 2005–2006 survey periods. Perhaps public health campaigns aimed at raising awareness of childhood over-weight were effective. Further data collection will reveal whether or not these rates reflect an actual plateau in the number of children becoming over-weight. As shown in **Figure 1.3**, the rate of in-crease in childhood obesity is slowing yet the num-ber of children who are at an unhealthy weight remains excessively high.

Severe Obesity in Children

Contrary to the general leveling trend, there are some weight category subgroups that are newly and rapidly increasing. The data showed that extreme obesity is no longer a disease that occurs only in adults; it is also increasingly seen in children (In a study of more than 700,000 patients age 2 to 19 years, 6.4% met the criteria for extreme childhood obesity (Koebnick, 2010). Another study showed that the group that includes the very heavi-est boys age 6 to 19 years seemed to be increasing the most (Ogden, 2010). There are also dramatic ethnic differences. Eleven percent of Hispanic boys and 12% of African-American girls were classified in the highest obesity category (Koebnick, 2010). These statistics raise great concern about the future health and well-being of American youth. It

is possible that these children will face the adverse health effects that come with obesity at a very early age. They are also likely to continue to be obese adults with consequences that potentially become more severe into middle and older ages.

BOX 1.1   Childhood Extreme Obesity

Childhood extreme obesity is defined as BMI-for-age equal to or greater than 120% of the 95th percentile. That equals a BMI of 35 or more (Skelton, 2009). A normal-weight 10-year-old child would weigh about 70 pounds. To be classified in the extreme obesity category, that child would weigh 140 pounds.

Disparities According to Sex and Ethnicity

A growing body of evidence suggests that inci-dence of obesity is influenced by social variables such as gender roles and ethnicity. The prevalence of obesity is increasing among all age and racial groups in the United States. There is, however, a disproportionate rise in the prevalence of obesity among blacks (African-Americans) and Mexican-Americans, especially in women, when compared to whites in the United States.

Table 1.2 displays NHANES data that indi-cates higher obesity prevalence for blacks and Mexican-Americans compared with non-Hispanic whites. While there are no NHANES estimates for other ethnic minority populations, alternate survey sources have shown that adult obesity prevalence is higher for American Indians, Alaska Natives, Native Hawaiians, and Pacific Islanders in comparison with non-Hispanic whites (Mullis, 2004). Immigrants to America have increased risk of overweight and obesity related to the length of time they live in the United States (Goel, 2004; Kaplan, 2004). Ethnicity-related disparity in obesity occurrence indicates that genetic factors are likely involved. Even so, exposure and responses

FIGURE **1.3**   Trends in childhood obesity in the United States, 1963–2008.

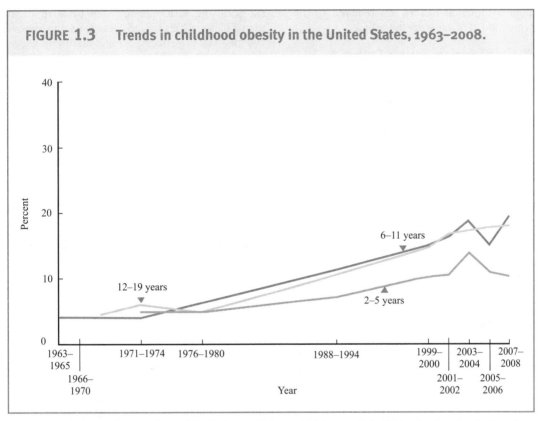

Source: Ogden C, Carroll M. Prevalence of Obesity Among Children and Adolescents: United States, Trends 1963-1965 Through 2007–2008, 2010; http://www.cdc.gov/nchs/data/hestat/obesity_child_07_08/obesity_child_07_08.pdf

TABLE **1.2**   Percentage Overweight and Obese According to Sex and Ethnicity: 2007–2008 NHANES Report

	Total	White*	Black**	Mexican-American
Overweight/obese	68			
Male	72	73	69	80
Female	64	61	78	77
Obese	34			
Male	32	32	37	36
Female	36	33	50	45

*Non-Hispanic white; **Non-Hispanic black
Adapted from: Flegal KM, Carroll MD, Ogden CL, Curtin LR. Prevalence and trends in obesity among US adults, 1999–2008. *JAMA*. Jan 20 2010;303(3):235–241.

to environmental factors are required to allow expression of obesity-related genes.

Effects of Socioeconomic Status

Nationwide surveys have traditionally shown a higher prevalence of obesity in populations with low SES. Patterns of SES differences are complex and not consistent across age, gender, and ethnicity. For example, in 2002 NHANES data, an inverse association of obesity prevalence with SES was observed in white girls, whereas higher SES was associated with higher obesity levels in African-American girls (Kumanyika, 2008). According to data from the National Survey of Children's Health, an increase in obesity is evident among children living in low-income, low-education, and higher-unemployment households. Children from these households had three to four times higher odds of being obese than children from higher socioeconomic households. The magnitude of socioeconomic disparities in obesity and overweight prevalence has steadily increased with large social inequalities persisting even after controlling for behavioral factors (Singh, 2010). Communities and individuals with low SES are at an evident disadvantage when it comes to healthy eating habits. The lower the income, the higher is the tendency towards a high-calorie, fast food diet. Access to low-cost healthful foods and opportunities for recreational physical activity have a major influence on weight and health (Drewnowski, 2009).

Global Trends

The rate of obesity is increasing around the world. The World Health Organization (WHO) monitors the global prevalence of obesity. Although obesity rates vary dramatically from nation to nation, the WHO estimates that more than 1.5 billion people are overweight. Of these, approximately 300 million women and 200 million men are obese. Rates of obesity have reached 20 to 30% in some European countries and over 70% in Polynesia. In a 2011 WHO report, the portion of the population who are obese in Nauru, a South Pacific island nation, is an astonishing 78.5% and it is nearly as high (74.6%) in American Samoa (WHO, 2011). The Middle East, Pacific Islands, Southeast Asia, and China are all facing serious challenges to control the rapid increase in obesity. Given these

statistics, the WHO projects that by 2015 more than 2 billion adults will be overweight and at least 700 million will be obese. There is enormous variation in obesity prevalence and progression within and between developed and developing countries. The WHO in its Global Database on BMI monitors the spectrum of weight and health status of the adult population worldwide. The database provides statistics about adult underweight, overweight, and obesity prevalence rates by country, year of survey, and sex. View this informative tool at the website listed in the Resources section of this chapter.

BOX 1.2   **Aims of the WHO Global Database on BMI**

- Monitor the spectrum of the nutritional status of adult population worldwide.
- Provide periodic updates of global, regional, and national prevalence rates and trends on underweight, overweight/obesity among adult populations.
- Report the global and regional estimated number of underweight, overweight, and obese adults.
- Identify vulnerable population groups (i.e., age, sex, geographical area).
- Assess the trends in nutrition transition (i.e., relationship between BMI and dietary patterns).
- Contribute to the identification and evaluation of intervention programs.
- Raise political awareness and commitment for action.

Courtesy of: WHO. About the BMI database. http://apps.who.int/bmi/index.jsp?introPage=intro_2.html.

Once considered a problem only in high-income countries, obesity is now on the rise in low- and middle-income countries, primarily in urban areas. In 2000 the number of people in the world who were obese outnumbered people suffering from undernutrition. In many countries economic development results in a nutrition transition where undernutrition coexists with obesity. Beneficial economic developments, such as increased wealth, better healthcare, and a reduced need for subsistence farming, have led to increased rates of obesity for some even when the number of hungry people remains high. Developing countries also face a "double burden" of disease. Infectious diseases and hunger exist side by side with diseases of obesity and overweight within the same country or even within the same household (Gardner, 2000). A 2006 study showed that the majority of India's citizens were undernourished, yet a growing segment of wealthy Indians was becoming obese (Subramanian, 2006). Previously, obesity in developing countries primarily affected the wealthy people who had access to plentiful food. Now there are growing levels of obesity among those of lower-income status as cheap, high-fat and high-sugar foods have become widely available. In 1989 national surveys in Brazil found that obesity in adults was more prevalent in the higher socioeconomic levels. Ten years later the lower socioeconomic group had a higher percentage of obese individuals (Caballero, 2007). This demographic switch foretells that the developing world may have to cope with the health problems of populations moving from hunger to obesity in a single generation.

Childhood Overweight Is Not Unique to the United States

More than 10% of the world's children in both developed and developing nations are overweight or obese. Even the youngest children are affected.

Twenty-two million children throughout the world younger than age 5 are overweight (WHO, 2011). In 2005, Wang and colleagues reported that 20% of Chinese children between ages 7 and 17 years who lived in large cities fell into the overweight category (Wang, 2005). In Europe childhood obesity is most prevalent in Southern European countries. International Obesity Task Force (IOTF) researchers surveying that region reported in 2004 that more than a third of 9-year-olds in mainland Italy and Sicily and 27% of children and adolescents in Spain were overweight or obese. In Crete, nearly 40% of children age 12 were overweight (Lobstein, 2004).

Summary

Trend surveys show that obesity is a serious public health challenge in the United States and internationally in both developed and developing countries. Over the past few decades the occurrence of obesity in adults and children has dramatically increased. Two-thirds of all American adults are overweight and a third of that group is obese (Flegal, 2010). In school-aged children and adolescents 32% are overweight including 17% who are categorized as obese (Ogden, 2010). The BMI distribution is becoming skewed, as the lower levels have remained fairly stable while the range of BMI values above 30 has widened substantially. Complex disparities in obesity susceptibility exist among men and women and among various ethnic and socioeconomic groups in the United States and throughout the world. An important individual and public health goal to reverse these trends would be to focus on realistic treatment and prevention strategies.

Critical Thinking Questions

Question: What is your state's obesity rate? What are some explanations for why obesity varies geographically in the United States?

Question: Do you think the plateau in the prevalence of obesity in 2010 is a result of beneficial effects of public health programs to control the problem or perhaps that the segment of the population who was susceptible to obesity had already become obese?

Resources

Public Health Agencies and Organizations That Monitor Obesity and Related Diseases

Centers for Disease Control and Prevention

http://www.cdc.gov/

Weight-control Information Network

http://www.win.niddk.nih.gov/

National Center for Health Statistics (http://www.cdc.gov/nchs/)

World Health Organization

http://www.who.int/en/

Obesity Trends Websites

Obesity by Race/Ethnicity 2006–2008

http://www.cdc.gov/nchs/data/hestat/obesity_adult_07_08/obesity_adult_07_08.htm\

United States Percent Prevalence of Overweight and Obesity and Trends by State 1985–2010

http://www.cdc.gov/obesity/data/trends.html

WHO Global Database on Body Mass Index

http://apps.who.int/bmi/

This tool presents BMI data interactively as maps, tables, graphs, and downloadable documents.

References

Benjamin R. The Surgeon General's Vision for a Healthy and Fit Nation 2010. Rockville, MD: Department of Health and Human Services Office of the Surgeon General; 2010.

Caballero B. The global epidemic of obesity: an overview. *Epidemiol Rev.* 2007;29:1–5.

CDC. Centers for Disease Control and Prevention. Behavioral Risk Factor Surveillance System Survey Data Trends 1976–1980 Through 2007–2008. 2010; http://www.cdc.gov/nchs/data/hestat/obesity_adult_07_08/obesity_adult_07_08.htm.

CDC. Centers for Disease Control and Prevention. Basics About Childhood Obesity. 2010; http://www.cdc.gov/obesity/childhood/defining.html. Accessed July 15, 2011.

Daniels SR, Arnett DK, Eckel RH, et al. Overweight in children and adolescents: pathophysiology, consequences, prevention, and treatment. *Circulation.* Apr 19 2005;111(15):1999–2012.

Drewnowski A. Obesity, diets, and social inequalities. *Nutr Rev.* May 2009;67 Suppl 1:S36–S39.

Flegal KM, Carroll MD, Ogden CL, Curtin LR. Prevalence and trends in obesity among US adults, 1999–2008. *JAMA.* Jan 20 2010;303(3):235–241.

Gardner G, Halweil B. *Overfed and Underfed: The Global Epidemic of Malnutrition.* Washington, DC: Worldwatch Institute; 2000.

Goel MS, McCarthy EP, Phillips RS, Wee CC. Obesity among US immigrant subgroups by duration of residence. *JAMA.* Dec 15 2004;292(23):2860–2867.

Kaplan MS, Huguet N, Newsom JT, McFarland BH. The association between length of residence and obesity among Hispanic immigrants. *Am J Prev Med.* Nov 2004;27(4):323–326.

Koebnick C, Smith N, Coleman KJ, et al. Prevalence of extreme obesity in a multiethnic cohort of children and adolescents. *J Pediatr.* Jul 2010;157(1):26–31, e22.

Kumanyika SK, Obarzanek E, Stettler N, et al. Population-based prevention of obesity: the need for comprehensive promotion of healthful eating, physical activity, and energy balance: a scientific statement from American Heart Association Council on Epidemiology and Prevention, Interdisciplinary Committee for Prevention (formerly the expert panel on population and prevention science). *Circulation.* Jul 22, 2008;118(4):428–464.

Lobstein T, Baur L, Uauy R. Obesity in children and young people: a crisis in public health. *Obes Rev.* May 2004; 5 Suppl 1:4–104.

Mullis RM, Blair SN, Aronne LJ, et al. Prevention Conference VII: obesity, a worldwide epidemic related to heart disease and stroke: Group IV: prevention/treatment. *Circulation.* Nov 2 2004;110(18):e484–e488.

NCHS. National Center for Health Statistics. Prevalence of Overweight, Infants and Children Less Than 2 Years of Age: United States, 2003–2004. *National Center for Health Statistics.* 2010; http://www.cdc.gov/nchs/data/hestat/overweight/overweight_child_under02.htm. Accessed January 2011.

Ogden CL, Carroll MD, Curtin LR, Lamb MM, Flegal KM. Prevalence of high body mass index in US children and adolescents, 2007–2008. *JAMA.* Jan 20 2010; 303(3):242–249.

Singh GK, Siahpush M, Kogan MD. Rising social inequalities in US childhood obesity, 2003–2007. *Ann Epidemiol.* Jan 2010;20(1):40–52.

Skelton JA, Cook SR, Auinger P, Klein JD, Barlow SE. Prevalence and trends of severe obesity among US children and adolescents. *Acad Pediatr.* Sep–Oct 2009;9(5):322–329.

Stewart ST, Cutler DM, Rosen AB. Forecasting the effects of obesity and smoking on U.S. life expectancy. *N Engl J Med.* Dec 3 2009;361(23):2252–2260.

Sturm R. Increases in clinically severe obesity in the United States, 1986–2000. *Arch Intern Med.* Oct 13 2003;163(18):2146–2148.

Subramanian SV, Smith GD. Patterns, distribution, and determinants of under- and overnutrition: a population-based study of women in India. *Am J Clin Nutr.* Sep 2006;84(3):633–640.

Wang L, Kong L, Wu F, Bai Y, Burton R. Preventing chronic diseases in China. *Lancet.* Nov 19 2005;366(9499): 1821–1824.

WHO. World Health Organization. Obesity and Overweight Fact Sheet No. 311. 2011; http://www.who.int/mediacentre/factsheets/fs311/en/. Accessed March 20, 2011.

CHAPTER 2

ASSESSMENT OF BODY WEIGHT AND BODY COMPOSITION

READER OBJECTIVES

- Describe typical anthropometric measures to assess body weight
- Define body mass index (BMI)
- Using BMI, distinguish among healthy weight, overweight, and obesity
- Describe the assessment of body composition including appropriate methodologies for adults
- Indicate the importance of waist circumference assessment and describe waist measurement techniques
- Interpret variations in BMI according to body composition, sex, and ethnicity
- Consider the significance of other disease conditions or risk factors when assessing overweight and obesity
- Compare obesity assessment for children and teens with adult evaluations

CHAPTER OUTLINE

Anthropometric Assessment of Optimal Body Weight

Anthropometric Assessment of Optimal Body Weight

The **anthropometric** assessment and definition of optimal weight, overweight, and obesity is somewhat subjective and imprecise. Overweight is generally defined as having more body weight than is considered healthy for one's age, sex, or height. The term *obese* is applied to overweight people who have a high percentage of body fat. Optimal weights have been variously referred to as ideal, desirable, or healthy. In addition to these subjective terms there are several types of objective criteria to define various levels of weight status.

Height-Weight Tables

Weight status can be assessed with height-weight tables such as those developed by the Metropolitan Life Insurance Company (MLIC). These tables of weight-for-height consider sex and frame size to determine a desirable weight associated with greater life expectancy. In 1942 a statistician at the MLIC grouped several million people who were insured with Metropolitan Life into categories based on their height, body frame (small, medium, or large), and weight. He discovered that the ones who lived the longest were the ones who maintained their body weight at the level that was the average for 25-year-olds. The results were published in tables and became widely used for determining "ideal" body weights over the next four decades. In 1983 the tables were revised and called simply "height and weight" tables without any "desirable weight" or "ideal weight" designations. They became the accepted guides for a healthy weight that were used by both the public and clinicians for decades. Healthy weight goals for men and women suggested by the MLIC in 1983 are shown in **Tables 2.1**. To determine whether a person is small, medium, or large boned based on wrist measurement, use the instructions in **Table 2.2** (see **Figure 2.1**).

Questions exist about the suitability of these tables to determine appropriate body weights because the suggested weights were based on incomplete or unbalanced measurements of a group of individuals that did not necessary reflect the general population. Examples of controversial issues include:

- The tables were based on a predominantly white, middle-class population.
- Some individuals were actually weighed and some reported their estimated weight.
- Height and weight was measured in people wearing shoes and clothing of varying amounts.
- Frame size was not consistently measured.
- Both smokers and nonsmokers were included. Smoking affects health as much as weight.

Experts suggest that height-weight tables may be used as a rough guide; however, additional factors including family history, level of physical activity, smoking and dietary habits, and body fat distribution should be included for a more complete evaluation of an individual's health risks (NHLBI, 1998).

Calculating Ideal Body Weight

A quick, easy calculation for **ideal body weight (IBW)** is often used as part of health risk assessment in clinical situations. The Hamwi formulas developed in 1964 are simple equations to determine IBW.

••

The formulas for IBW are:

Men: 106 lb for the first 5 ft; 6 lb for each inch over 5 ft
Women: 100 lb for the first 5 ft; 5 lb for each inch over 5 ft

In addition, a range of 10% variation above or below the calculated weight is allowed for individual differences.

Example:
Estimate ideal body weight of a man who is 5 ft 10 in. tall.

$$106 + (6 \times 10) = 106 + 60 = 166 \text{ lb}$$

The IBW range with 10% variation below and above is 149 to 183 lb.

$$(10\% \text{ of } 166 = \text{about } 17 \text{ lb; so } 166 - 17 = 149$$
$$\text{and } 166 + 17 = 183)$$

Estimate ideal body weight of a woman who is 5 ft 10 in. tall.

$$100 + (5 \times 10) = 100 + 50 = 150 \text{ lb}$$

TABLE 2.1   1983 Metropolitan Height and Weight Tables

	Weight Chart for Women				Weight Chart for Men		
Height	**Small frame**	**Medium frame**	**Large frame**	**Height**	**Small frame**	**Medium frame**	**Large frame**
4'10"	102–111	109–121	118–131	5'2"	128–134	131–141	138–150
4'11"	103–113	111–123	120–134	5'3"	130–136	133–143	140–153
5'0"	104–115	113–126	122–137	5'4"	132–138	135–145	142–156
5'1"	106–118	115–129	125–140	5'5"	134–140	137–148	144–160
5'2"	108–121	118–132	128–143	5'6"	136–142	139–151	146–164
5'3"	111–124	121–135	131–147	5'7"	138–145	142–154	149–168
5'4"	114–127	124–138	134–151	5'8"	140–148	145–157	152–172
5'5"	117–130	127–141	137–155	5'9"	142–151	148–160	155–176
5'6"	120–133	130–144	140–159	5'10"	144–154	151–163	158–180
5'7"	123–136	133–147	143–163	5'11"	146–157	154–166	161–184
5'8"	126–139	136–150	146–167	6'0"	149–160	157–170	164–188
5'9"	129–142	139–153	149–170	6'1"	152–164	160–174	168–192
5'10"	132–145	142–156	152–173	6'2"	155–168	164–178	172–197
5'11"	135–148	145–159	155–176	6'3"	158–172	167–182	176–202
6'0"	138–151	148–162	158–179	6'4"	162–176	171–187	181–207

Weight in pounds, based on ages 25–59 with the lowest mortality rate (indoor clothing weighing 3 lb and shoes with 1-in. heels)

Weight in pounds, based on ages 25–59 with the lowest mortality rate (indoor clothing weighing 5 lb and shoes with 1-in. heels)

Adapted from: Metropolitan height and weight standards. *Statistical Bulletin of New York Metlife Insurance Company.* Vol 64: Metropolitan Life Insurance Company; 1983:2–9.

The IBW range with 10% variation below and above is 135 to 165 lb.

$$(10\% \text{ of } 150 = 15 \text{ lb}; \text{ so } 150 - 15 = 135$$
$$\text{and } 150 + 15 = 165)$$

••

While these calculations allow a rapid estimate of the range for a healthy body weight, criticisms of the IBW formula are that it does not correlate weight to health or prevention of disease or make allowance for body composition or body type. For example, a person with a large frame size or with a high percentage of lean muscle would appear to be overweight according to this method.

Comprehensive and Consistent Assessment of Overweight and Obesity Recommended by National Institutes of Health (NIH)

To help healthcare professionals select efficient, appropriate, and evidence-based methods to assess and manage overweight and obesity and to alert practitioners about health risks associated

TABLE 2.2	Using Wrist Measurement to Determine Frame Size Measurement for Women and Men

To determine the body frame size, measure the wrist and use the results to assess whether the person is small, medium, or large boned.

Women

Height under 5'2"

- Small = wrist size less than 5.5"
- Medium = wrist size 5.5" to 5.75"
- Large = wrist size over 5.75"

Height 5'2" to 5'5"

- Small = wrist size less than 6"
- Medium = wrist size 6" to 6.25"
- Large = wrist size over 6.25"

Height over 5'5"

- Small = wrist size less than 6.25"
- Medium = wrist size 6.25" to 6.5"
- Large = wrist size over 6.5"

Men

Height over 5'5"

- Small = wrist size 5.5" to 6.5"
- Medium = wrist size 6.5" to 7.5"
- Large = wrist size over 7.5"

Source: © 2012 A.D.A.M., Inc.

with obesity, the *Clinical Guidelines on the Identification, Evaluation, and Treatment of Overweight and Obesity in Adults* was released by the National Heart, Lung, and Blood Institute's (NHLBI) Obesity Education Initiative Expert Panel in 1998. For details about how the guidelines were developed and to see the "Ten Steps to Treating Overweight and Obesity in the Primary Care Setting" check the website listed in the Resources section at the end of this chapter.

Because obesity is associated with an increased risk of a variety of diseases and health problems, the NHLBI expert panel recommends evaluation of obesity-related health risk using three measures:

- Determine BMI.
- Evaluate fat distribution using waist circumference measurement.
- Assess other health risk factors and presence of obesity-related diseases.

How Is BMI Useful?

For appraisal of health risk associated with obesity, the NHLBI expert panel uses the body mass index or BMI. BMI is a mathematical calculation based on height and weight, and it is the same for both sexes and for all adults without regard to age or ethnicity. While the BMI calculation is an indirect measurement, it has been shown to be a fairly reliable measure of degree of body fat in the general population. It also is a practical indicator of the severity of obesity.

Calculating BMI

BMI can be calculated in a two ways:

Using kilograms and meters: Weight in kilograms divided by height in meters squared.

Example: Weight = 70 kg, Height = 166 cm (1.66 m) BMI Calculation: $70/(1.66)^2 = 25.3$ kg/m^2*

Using pounds and inches: weight in pounds divided by height in inches squared × 703.

Example: Weight = 140 lb, Height = 5 ft 5 in. (65 in.) BMI Calculation: $[140/(65)^2] \times 703 = 23.3$*

How to convert pounds to kilograms and inches to centimeters:

Weight in pounds _____ divide by 2.2 = _____ kilograms (kg)
Height in inches _____ multiply by 2.54 = _____ centimeters (cm)

***Note:** In scientific papers BMI is reported with kg/m^2 as the units. Throughout this text only the BMI number will be reported without the unit identification (e.g., BMI = 25).
Hint: No calculations are needed to find BMI in a table or an online BMI calculator.

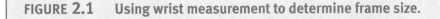

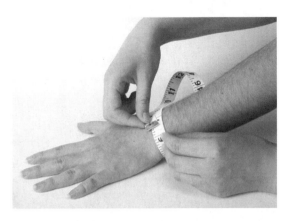

FIGURE 2.1   Using wrist measurement to determine frame size.

Source: © Jones & Bartlett Learning. Photo by Amy Rathburn.

Look at the BMI table in **Figure 2.2** or try the online BMI calculators listed in the Resources section at the end of the chapter. To use the BMI table, find the appropriate height in the left-hand column. Move across the row to the given weight. The number at the top of the column is the BMI for that height and weight.

BMI Categories

The classification of overweight and obesity, based on the measurement of BMI, is primarily designed to assess risk of disease. In 1998 the NHLBI expert panel report used the BMI range of 19–24.9 as the basis for defining healthy weights for adults. The definition of overweight as a BMI equal to or greater than (≥) 25 is justified with evidence that showed increased **morbidity** and **mortality** occurred at BMI greater than 25. Given individual variability, it is difficult to assign a specific BMI that is associated with increased health risk. For example, if a person is considered to be healthy at a normal BMI of 24.5, is there an absolute health risk increase at 25.5? With this ambiguity in mind, the NHLBI recommended use of a figure with shaded BMI category areas to reflect the uncertainty of risk cutoffs for increasing levels of overweight above a BMI of 25 (NHLBI, 1998). For general assessment, an adult who has a BMI between 25 and 29.9 is

considered overweight and obesity is defined as a BMI ≥ 30. These definitions are widely used by the federal government, scientific and medical communities, and the public. See the BMI categories in **Table 2.3**.

The World Health Organization provided refinements to the classification system that included three grades of overweight using BMI cutoff points of 25, 30, and 40, as shown in **Table 2.4**. Further modifications to these definitions have been suggested. Studies and literature related to obesity surgery define obesity in categories of severity. With the increase in the number of people in the higher BMI categories, these extended classes may become more useful (Sturm, 2007):

- BMI 40 to 44.9 is severe obesity.
- BMI 45 to 49.9 is morbid obesity.
- BMI ≥ 50 is super obese.

BMI Variation According to Ethnicity

As obesity is defined as a condition related to excess body fat, accumulating evidence has suggested that the relationship between BMI and degree of fatness differs among ethnic groups. The interpretation of BMI grades relative to disease risk may differ as a result. Experts with the WHO have concluded that increases in health-related

FIGURE 2.2 Body mass index table.

Body Weight (pounds)

Height (inches) \ BMI	19	20	21	22	23	24	25	26	27	28	29	30	31	32	33	34	35	36	37	38	39	40	41	42	43	44	45	46	47	48	49	50	51	52	53	54
58	91	96	100	105	110	115	119	124	129	134	138	143	148	153	158	162	167	172	177	181	186	191	196	201	205	210	215	220	224	229	234	239	244	248	253	258
59	94	99	104	109	114	119	124	128	133	138	143	148	153	158	163	168	173	178	183	188	193	198	203	208	212	217	222	227	232	237	242	247	252	257	262	267
60	97	102	107	112	118	123	128	133	138	143	148	153	158	163	168	174	179	184	189	194	199	204	209	215	220	225	230	235	240	245	250	255	261	266	271	276
61	100	106	111	116	122	127	132	137	143	148	153	158	164	169	174	180	185	190	195	201	206	211	217	222	227	232	238	243	248	254	259	264	269	275	280	285
62	104	109	115	120	126	131	136	142	147	153	158	164	169	175	180	186	191	196	202	207	213	218	224	229	235	240	246	251	256	262	267	273	278	284	289	295
63	107	113	118	124	130	135	141	146	152	158	163	169	175	180	186	191	197	203	208	214	220	225	231	237	242	248	254	259	265	270	278	282	287	293	299	304
64	110	116	122	128	134	140	145	151	157	162	169	174	180	186	192	197	204	209	215	221	227	232	238	244	250	256	262	267	273	279	285	291	296	302	308	314
65	114	120	126	132	138	144	150	156	162	168	174	180	186	192	198	204	210	216	222	228	234	240	246	252	258	264	270	276	282	288	294	300	306	312	318	324
66	118	124	130	136	142	148	155	161	167	173	179	186	192	198	204	210	216	223	229	235	241	247	253	260	266	272	278	284	291	297	303	309	315	322	328	334
67	121	127	134	140	146	153	159	166	172	178	185	191	198	204	211	217	223	230	236	242	249	255	261	268	274	280	287	293	299	306	312	319	325	331	338	344
68	125	131	138	144	151	158	164	171	177	184	190	197	203	210	216	223	230	236	243	249	256	262	269	276	282	289	295	302	308	315	322	328	335	341	348	354
69	128	135	142	149	155	162	169	176	182	189	196	203	209	216	223	230	236	243	250	257	263	270	277	284	291	297	304	311	318	324	331	338	345	351	358	365
70	132	139	146	153	160	167	174	181	188	195	202	209	216	222	229	236	243	250	257	264	271	278	285	292	299	306	313	320	327	334	341	348	355	362	369	376
71	136	143	150	157	165	172	179	186	193	200	208	215	222	229	236	243	250	257	265	272	279	286	293	301	308	315	322	329	338	343	351	358	365	372	379	386
72	140	147	154	162	169	177	184	191	199	206	213	221	228	235	242	250	258	265	272	279	287	294	302	309	316	324	331	338	346	353	361	368	375	383	390	397
73	144	151	159	166	174	182	189	197	204	212	219	227	235	242	250	257	265	272	280	288	295	302	310	318	325	333	340	348	355	363	371	378	386	393	401	408
74	148	155	163	171	179	186	194	202	210	218	225	233	241	249	256	264	272	280	287	295	303	311	319	326	334	342	350	358	365	373	381	389	396	404	412	420
75	152	160	168	176	184	192	200	208	216	224	232	240	248	256	264	272	279	287	295	303	311	319	327	335	343	351	359	367	375	383	391	399	407	415	423	431
76	156	164	172	180	189	197	205	213	221	230	238	246	254	263	271	279	287	295	304	312	320	328	336	344	353	361	369	377	385	394	402	410	418	426	435	443

Source: NHLBI. *Clinical Guidelines on the Identification, Evaluation, and Treatment of Overweight and Obesity in Adults—The Evidence Report.* National Institutes of Health, National Heart, Lung, and Blood Institute. September 1998: http://www.nhlbi.nih.gov/guidelines/obesity/bmi_tbl.htm.

TABLE 2.3	Example of Weight Ranges Compared with BMI Values Used to Determine Underweight, Healthy Weight, or Overweight		
Height	**Weight range**	**BMI**	**Health category**
5'9"	124 lb or less	Below 18.5	Underweight
	125 lb to 168 lb	18.5 to 24.9	Healthy weight
	169 lb to 202 lb	25.0 to 29.9	Overweight
	203 lb or more	30 or higher	Obese

This example is for a person 5 ft 9 in. tall.
Courtesy of: the Centers for Disease Control and Prevention.

TABLE 2.4	World Health Organization BMI Categories
Classification	**BMI (kg/m²)**
	Principal cutoff points
Normal range	18.50–24.99
Overweight	≥ 25.00
Pre-obese	25.00–29.99
Obese	≥ 30.00
Obese class I	30.00–34.99
Obese class II	35.00–39.99
Obese class III	≥ 40.00

Reproduced from: The International Classification of adult underweight, overweight and obesity according to BMI http://apps.who.int/bmi/index.jsp?introPage=intro_3.html

risk factors and comorbidities associated with obesity occur at a lower BMI in Asian populations than in other ethnic groups (WHO, 2004). Possible explanations for these differences might be variations in activity level, body proportions, frame size, and in muscle mass versus fat mass (Deurenberg, 2002). For example, Pacific Islanders appear to be more muscular and have lower levels of body fat at a given BMI. In the United States, African-Americans have been shown to have fewer health-related risk factors at a given BMI. Experts have suggested that overweight and obesity may have to be redefined for some populations. On the basis of the respective health-related risk factors and comorbidities, lower cutoff points for Asians were identified for overweight (BMI ≥ 23.0) and obesity (BMI ≥ 25.0) and cutoff points higher than a BMI of 30 in Pacific Islanders (Hubbard, 2000) and American blacks (Deurenberg, 2002) were advised. Alternate BMI cutoff values could be used for public health action and for reporting purposes in international comparisons. Highlighting the variation in BMI-related health consequences according to ethnicity is noteworthy in that it brings into focus a broad international perspective on the association of ethnicity and disease risk (WHO, 2004).

BMI Limitations

BMI is frequently used in population studies because of its ease of determination and well-supported association with mortality and health effects. However, it should be considered as only a rough guide because it may not correspond to the same degree of fatness in different individuals. Even though the correlation between body fat measurement and BMI is fairly strong, the index does not directly measure body fat and it has some limitations based on differences in sex, age, ethnicity, and athletic experience. These limitations include the following:

- Women tend to have more body fat than men.
- BMI overestimates body fat in persons who are very muscular, placing them in an overweight or obese category when they are not overly fat.
- BMI can underestimate body fat in persons who have lost muscle mass (e.g., the elderly).
- BMI outside the healthy range without other risk factors may not indicate inappropriate body weight.

Despite these limitations it is usually assumed that people above optimal weight-for-height are over-fat as well as overweight. However, the fact that BMI does not convey information about fat distribution emphasizes the idea that the BMI category should serve as a generalized guideline and further assessment should be performed to reach a more complete view of individual health.

Assessment of Body Composition and Fat Distribution

BMI is not a specific index of fatness because its numerator—the measured body weight—reflects muscle, bone, and body water in addition to fat. State of hydration can make a large difference in BMI because drinking 16 oz of a beverage will increase body weight 1 lb (until it is excreted). Another example of variation in body weight composition is that very athletic persons may have a heavy body weight due to large amounts of muscle or lean body mass rather than excess body fat or **adipose tissue**. There are several different methods of assessing the percentage of fat and lean mass of an individual. These methods are referred to as **body composition** analysis. The various methods include water or air displacement, dual energy X-ray absorptiometry, bioelectrical impedance, and skinfold thickness measures.

Air and Water Displacement Techniques
Underwater Weighing
Underwater weighing, also known as hydrodensitometry or hydrostatic weighing, has been the

reference standard for assessing the relative amounts of fat and lean that make up body composition (see **Figure 2.3**). This technique involves weighing a person on dry land, and then reweighing when the individual is totally submerged in a tub of water. It is based on Archimedes's principle, which states that given an equal weight, lower-density objects have a larger surface area and displace more water than higher-density objects. Bone and muscle are denser than water and fat is less dense than water. In two individuals of the same weight but with different proportions of fat and lean, the one with the most body fat would displace more water. The volume of water displaced by the person and the difference between the dry weight

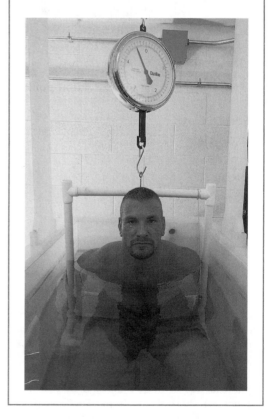

FIGURE 2.3   Underwater weighing.

and the submerged weight is entered into equations than can be used to estimate percentage of body fat. Disadvantages of this method are the cost and time required. It also relies on the participant's ability to fully exhale air in the lungs and to stay completely underwater during the measurement.

Air Displacement Plethysmography (ADP)

ADP is similar to hydrodensitometry; however, body volume is determined by displacement of air instead of water (see **Figure 2.4**). Pressure changes are measured when a subject sits in a small sealed chamber in which there is a known volume of air.

Large body volumes displace greater air volume and results in a larger increase in pressure in the chamber. Studies have demonstrated that both underwater weighing and ADP give similar body fat percentage results (Ellis, 2001). This technique has advantages over hydrodensitometry in that the participant does not have to control breathing and go underwater.

Dual Energy X-ray Absorptiometry (DEXA)

DEXA is a highly accurate way to assess body fat, although it is expensive and is generally limited to

FIGURE 2.4   Air displacement plethysmography BOD POD.

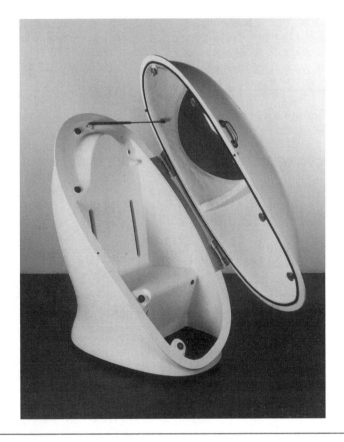

Courtesy of: COSMED USA, Inc.

clinical research studies. This method was originally developed to evaluate bone mineral density with a scanner that measures body composition using low-energy X-rays. As two X-ray beams pass through the individual, the amount of X-ray absorbed by the tissue reveals differences in fat from lean mass. The tissues with greater density (bone and muscle) show a greater reduction in X-ray that is allowed to pass through them. The level of radiation is low enough that DEXA is approved by the FDA as a screening device to predict body composition. It would take approximately 800 full-body DEXA scans to equal the amount of exposure to radiation received from one standard chest X-ray (Bolanowski, 2001).

Bioelectrical Impedance Analysis (BIA)

BIA is another method of assessing body fat percentage (see **Figure 2.5**). BIA is based on the principle that body tissue is capable of conducting electricity. Water is a good conductor of electricity, and most body water is found in lean tissue. Fat is a poor conductor of electricity and it slows down, or impedes, the electrical flow. A high-resistance measurement signals a high level of fat. As the BIA method is population specific and the validity is influenced by sex, age, disease state, race, or ethnicity, impedance is calculated by entering the resistance data into equations specific to the population being measured. This analyzer was developed as a lab device for research studies that involved attaching electrodes to the hands and feet and, with the subject resting and supine, the total body electrical impedance or resistance was measured. Under controlled conditions and using the appropriate equations, accuracy of this method to estimate body fat is 4 to 7% (Lee, 2008). There are now a variety of body composition and body fat analyzers and scales available for home use that determine total body water, fat, and muscle mass.

BIA is considered to be safe because BIA currents (at a frequency of 50 kHz) are not noticeable and are unlikely to affect tissues, such as nerves or cardiac muscle that could be susceptible to electric

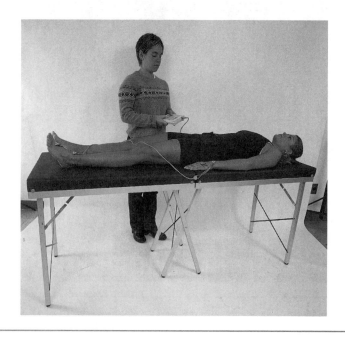

FIGURE **2.5**   Bioelectrical impedance analysis (BIA).

stimulation. However, anyone with an implanted defibrillator should avoid BIA evaluation because even low currents could potentially provoke an inappropriate defibrillator response (NHLBI, 1998). BIA has some limitations, as it is very sensitive to hydration levels, food intake, skin temperature, and recent exercise. The advantages of BIA include its ease of use, relatively low cost, portability, and the fact that minimal participant participation is required.

Skinfold Measurement

Body density estimation from skinfold measurement has the advantages of simplicity, low cost, and reasonable validity. Predictions for most individuals fall within 3 to 4% of measures that would be determined with hydrodensitometry. The technique is based on the assumption that **subcutaneous fat** will be a representation of the total fat content of the body. Precision calipers are used to measure subcutaneous fat at specific sites around the body including the chest, hip, abdomen, thigh, and upper arm. The sum of these measures is entered into prediction equations to estimate total body fat. The choice of prediction equation will depend on whether a generalized equation or a population-specific equation is appropriate. Body density and percentage of body fat can also be determined by entering skinfold measurement values into calculators on skinfold measurement websites. The Resources section provides websites for skinfold measurement techniques and calculators.

Additional advantages of skinfold testing are that it is fast, portable, and easy for the individual being assessed. When using skinfold assessment, it is assumed that:

- About 50% of fat is subcutaneous.
- The testing sites represent an average thickness of all subcutaneous fat.
- Compressibility of fat will be similar among subjects.
- The thickness of skin is negligible.

Although skinfold measurement is easily administered and practical, the technique does have limitations and relies on tester skill and other factors. Skinfold thickness may be reduced by dehydration or increased by exercise or **edema**. Limitations

on how wide the calipers open can make skinfold measurement challenging to use with extremely obese patients. In addition, not all body fat, such as abdominal fat, is accessible to the calipers, and the distribution of subcutaneous fat can vary significantly over the human body (Wang, 2000).

What Is a Normal Body Fat Percentage?

Epidemiologic studies show that levels of body fat associated with good health vary according to sex and age. While there are no universally accepted standards to describe optimal percentages, experts consider that an average amount of body fat is 12 to 24% for men and 20 to 30% for women. Any amount over that range would be a sign of obesity and increased risk for chronic disease (Abernathy, 1996; ACE, 2008). Although body fat amounts among elite athletes varies by sport, athletes tend to be at the low end of the scale because of their increased muscle mass. Generalized ranges for percentage of body fat are appropriate for use as screening tests but are not useful as strict guidelines for individuals.

Is Waist Circumference Measurement Better at Assessing Risk Than BMI?

Excessive abdominal or **visceral fat** tissue is associated with increased health risk compared with subcutaneous fat or fat distribution around the hips and thighs (Poirier, 2006). Waist circumference measurement can be used as an estimate for abdominal fat distribution and may be a better indicator of health risk than BMI alone. Waist circumference measurement can be particularly useful for further health appraisal in patients who are categorized as overweight on the BMI scale as there is an increased risk for type 2 diabetes, dyslipidemia, hypertension, and cardiovascular disease (CVD) in women with a waist circumference of more than 35 in. and men with a waist circumference of more than 40 in. no matter what the BMI value. Accordingly, the NHLBI clinical guidelines recommend the use of waist circumference in addition to BMI in clinical screening of adults (NHLBI, 1998). See how BMI and waist circumference are both associated with disease risk in **Table 2.5**.

Waist circumference cut points can generally be applied to all adult ethnic groups.

TABLE 2.5 Classification of Overweight and Obesity by BMI, Waist Circumference, and Associated Disease Risk*.

	BMI (kg/m²)	Obesity class	Waist circumference Men ≤102 cm (≤40 in.) Women ≤88 cm (≤35 in.)	Waist circumference Men >102 cm (>40 in.) Women >88 cm (>35 in.)
Underweight	< 18.5		—	—
Normal†	18.5 – 24.9		—	—
Overweight	25.0 – 29.9		Increased	High
Obese	30.0 – 34.9	I	High	Very high

*Disease risk for type 2 diabetes, hypertension, and CVD.
†Increased waist circumference can also be a marker for increased risk even in persons of normal weight.
Reproduced from: The Practical Guide to the Identification, Evaluation, and Treatment of Overweight and Obesity in Adults. National Heart, Lung, and Blood Institute and North American Association for the Study of Obesity. Bethesda, Md: National Institutes of Health; 2000. NIH Publication number 00-4084, October 2000. Adapted from Preventing and Managing the Global Epidemic of Obesity. Report of the World Health Organization Consultation of Obesity. WHO, Geneva, June 1997.

BOX 2.1 Waist Circumference Risk Categories

Men greater than or equal to 102 cm (40 in.)
Women greater than or equal to 88 cm (35 in.)

Reproduced from: The Practical Guide to the Identification, Evaluation, and Treatment of Overweight and Obesity in Adults. National Heart, Lung, and Blood Institute and North American Association for the Study of Obesity. Bethesda, Md: National Institutes of Health; 2000. NIH Publication number 00-4084, October 2000.

However, the World Health Organization reports that lower thresholds for waist circumference may be necessary for certain Asian populations. Those at increased risk for developing chronic disease include (WHO, 2004):

- Asian women with a waist circumference of more than 31 in.
- Asian men with a waist circumference of more than 35 in.

As shown in **Figure 2.6** waist circumference is measured just above the iliac crest or hip bone.

BOX 2.2 Other Terms That Describe Body Fat Distribution

Android Obesity
Abdominal obesity
Central obesity
Upper body fat
"Apple shape" obesity

Gynoid Obesity
Lower body obesity
"Pear shaped" obesity

Adapted from: The Practical Guide to the Identification, Evaluation, and Treatment of Overweight and Obesity in Adults. National Heart, Lung, and Blood Institute and North American Association for the Study of Obesity. Bethesda, Md: National Institutes of Health; 2000. NIH Publication number 00-4084, October 2000.

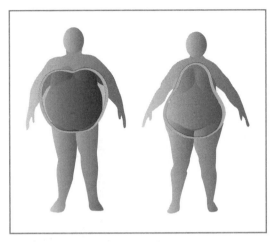

Presence of Other Risk Factors or Disease Comorbidities

Although disease risk generally increases with increasing BMI, susceptibility to metabolic abnormalities of comorbidities at a given weight varies among individuals. Having a BMI in the overweight or obese range does not necessarily indicate that a person is unhealthy. In fact, some individuals with a BMI less than 25 can have all the health consequences of overweight and obesity, whereas others may have fewer health issues with a higher BMI. Other risk factors, such as high blood pressure, high cholesterol, smoking, type 2 diabetes, medications, fitness level, and personal and family medical history are important considerations when assessing overall health (NHLBI, 1998).

FIGURE 2.6 **Measuring tape position for waist (abdominal) circumference.**

Modified from: The Practical Guide to the Identification, Evaluation, and Treatment of Overweight and Obesity in Adults. National Heart, Lung, and Blood Institute and North American Association for the Study of Obesity. Bethesda, MD: National Institutes of Health; 2000. NIH Publication number 00-4084, October 2000. http://www.nhlbi.nih.gov/guidelines/obesity/e_txtbk/txgd/4142.htm.

BOX 2.3 **Each Additional Risk Factor Increases Chronic Disease Risk**

High blood pressure (hypertension)
High LDL-cholesterol
Low HDL-cholesterol
High triglycerides
High blood glucose
Family history of premature heart disease
Physical inactivity
Cigarette smoking

Data from: The Practical Guide to the Identification, Evaluation, and Treatment of Overweight and Obesity in Adults. National Heart, Lung, and Blood Institute and North American Association for the Study of Obesity. Bethesda, Md: National Institutes of Health; 2000. NIH Publication number 00-4084, October 2000.

A comprehensive strategy for the evaluation and treatment of overweight patients is presented in the NIH/NHLBI Treatment Algorithm. This algorithm, shown in **Figure 2.7**, depicts the step-by-step assessment for overweight and obesity and

FIGURE 2.7 Algorithm for the assessment and treatment of overweight and obesity. The algorithm depicts the NHLBI expert panel's treatment decision process, which provides a step-by-step approach to managing overweight and obese patients.

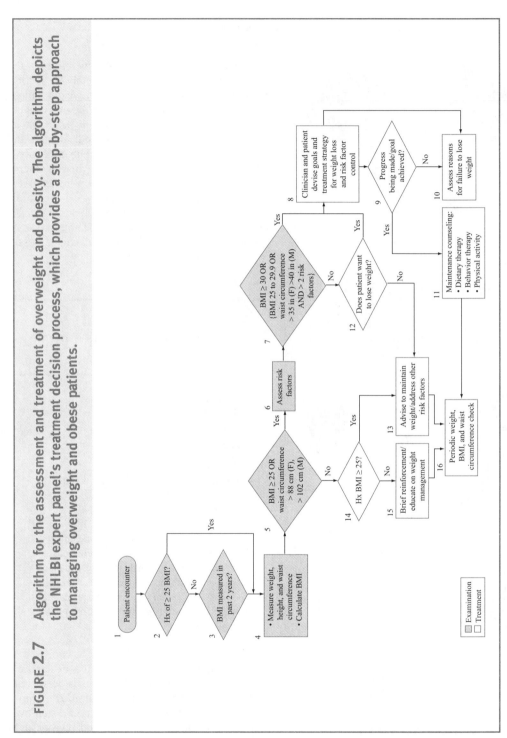

Source: The *Practical Guide to the Identification, Evaluation, and Treatment of Overweight and Obesity in Adults.* National Heart, Lung, and Blood Institute and North American Association for the Study of Obesity. Bethesda, MD: National Institutes of Health; 2000. NIH Publication number 00-4084, October 2000.

subsequent decisions based on that assessment. In overweight patients, management of all health risk factors deserves the same emphasis as weight-loss therapy. For example, reduction of other risk factors will reduce the possibility of acquiring cardiovascular disease or type 2 diabetes whether or not efforts at weight loss are successful.

Methods to Assess Childhood and Adolescent Overweight and Obesity

For anthropometric assessment, youth 6 to 17 years of age are classified as children, although the word *children* may also be applied to young-sters 6 to 11 years of age and *adolescents* may define individuals 12 to 17 years of age. BMI as a gauge of excess body fat is a less-effective mea-sure for children than for adults. A child's weight status is determined based on age- and sex-spe-cific percentiles for BMI rather than by the general BMI categories used for adults. Classifications of overweight and obesity for children and adoles-cents are based on growth rates and developmen-tal differences that vary between boys and girls. For these reasons, the BMI of a child is compared with the BMI of a reference population of children of the same sex and age. A child's BMI is plotted on CDC BMI-for-age growth charts specific for either girls or boys and the result is a percentile ranking. See **Table 2.6** for an example. The percentile indi-cates the relative position of the child's BMI among children of the same sex and age.

The definition of overweight or obesity for children has been controversial. In the past, the CDC has avoided the term *obese* when referring to body weight in children because of concerns about stigma and embarrassment for children and parents. In the United States overweight and obesity categories were described as "at risk for overweight" or "overweight" respectively. How-ever, for researchers and clinicians in the rest of the world a BMI-for-age at or above the 85th percentile is overweight and above the 95th per-centile is obese (Flodmark, 2004). These stan-dards, which linked children's BMI cutoffs to the accepted adult cutoff points of 25 and 30, were developed in 2000 by the International Associa-tion for the Study of Obesity (IASO). In 2007, an expert committee from the American Medical

TABLE 2.6	Children's BMI-for-Age Weight Status Categories
Weight status category	**Percentile range— compared with boys or girls of same age**
Underweight	Less than the 5th percentile
Healthy weight	5th percentile to less than the 85th percentile
At risk of overweight	85th percentile to less than the 95th percentile
Overweight	Equal to or greater than the 95th percentile

Courtesy of: the Centers for Disease Control and Prevention.

Association (AMA) recommended that the United States use similar terminology (Barlow, 2007). In addition, another category was proposed to define severe childhood obesity as BMI at or above the 99th percentile.

Since the release of the 2000 CDC growth charts, there has been a need to further classify extreme high values in children who are in the group above the 95th percentile of BMI-for-age. In adults, severe obesity (Class II with a BMI $\geq$ 35) corresponds to approximately 1.2 times the BMI 30 cut point to define obesity. Therefore, the proposed definition for extreme youth obesity was based on the threshold for childhood obesity. It is set at 1.2 times the 95th percentile of BMI-for-age or BMI $\geq$ 35 (Flegal, 2009).

Summary

Overweight and obesity are defined by excess body weight and body fat that may increase risk of chronic disease. Various tables and equations based on variables such as height, weight, sex, age, and frame size have been employed to iden-tify optimal weight. One commonly used measure is the body mass index (BMI). It is an index of weight-for-height used in classifying overweight and obesity in adults. Overweight is categorized by a BMI of 25 to 29.9 and obesity by a BMI of 30 or greater. While BMI is a good estimation of risk at the population level, it may not be as useful as a defining measure for individuals. BMI ranges for children and teens differ from adult categories, and they are defined so that they take into account normal differences in body fat between boys and girls and differences in body fat at various ages.

For most people, BMI correlates with degree of body fat. However, percentage of body fat does vary with individual body composition. The relationship between percentage of body fat and level of health risk associated with a particular BMI varies according to ethnic background. Methods to estimate body fat and body fat distribution include measurement of skinfold thickness, waist circumference, and more complicated techniques such as underwater weighing, bioelectrical impedance, and dual energy X-ray absorptiometry. In addition to anthropometric measures, experts advise that additional factors including family history, level of physical activity, and overall health and dietary habits should be included to evaluate an individual's health risk.

Critical Thinking Questions

Question: For evaluation of an individual's obesity-related health risk, what are three types of assessments that are recommended by the NHLBI *Clinical Guidelines on the Identification, Evaluation, and Treatment of Overweight and Obesity in Adults*? Give some specific examples of each type of assessment.

Question: Use the quick method to assess ideal body weight (IBW).

What would be the IBW for a male 5 ft 9 in. tall?

What would be the IBW for a female 5 ft 9 in. tall?

What factors account for the difference in IBW?

Question: Notice the difference in IBW for a man or a woman with the same height. What are some explanations about why the IBW varies with sex of the individual?

Question: Discuss how adding a measure of body fat distribution may help overcome limitations in health risk assessment associated with the single BMI measure.

Question: Two children have exactly the same BMI values. One is considered obese and the other is not. Why is that?

Activity: Check how childhood classifications change in various age groups using BMI-for-age growth charts on the CDC website.

Resources

Clinical Guidelines on the Identification, Evaluation, and Treatment of Overweight and Obesity in Adults
http://www.nhlbi.nih.gov/guidelines/obesity/index.htm

These guidelines provide the basic tools for assessing and managing obesity and also include practical information on dietary therapy, physical activity, and behavior therapy. There is also guidance on the appropriate use of pharmacotherapy and surgery as treatment options.

Obesity Definitions for Adults

http://www.cdc.gov/obesity/defining.html

Body Fat Percentage from Skinfold Measures

http://www.dietandfitnesstoday.com

Adult BMI Calculator

http://www.cdc.gov/healthyweight/assessing/bmi/adult_bmi/english_bmi_calculator/bmi_calculator.html

BMI Calculator for Adults and Children

http://www.cdc.gov/healthyweight/assessing/bmi/

BMI Percentile Calculator for Child and Teen

http://apps.nccd.cdc.gov/dnpaBMI/Calculator.aspx

This calculator provides BMI and the corresponding BMI-for-age percentile on a CDC BMI-for-age growth chart. Use this calculator for children and teens, age 2 to 19 years.

CDC Growth Chart Training Modules

http://www.cdc.gov/nccdphp/dnpao/growthcharts/training/modules.htm

Use these modules to learn more about how growth charts were developed and how to use them.

Childhood BMI Calculators and Tools from the USDA/ARS Children's Nutrition Research Center at Baylor College of Medicine

References

Abernathy RP, Black DR. Healthy body weights: an alternative perspective. *Am J Clin Nutr.* Mar 1996;63(3 Suppl):448S–451S.

ACE. American Council on Exercise Lifestyle & Weight Management Coach Manual. San Diego: American Council on Exercise; 2008.

Barlow SE. Expert committee recommendations regarding the prevention, assessment, and treatment of child and adolescent overweight and obesity: summary report. *Pediatrics.* Dec 2007;120 Suppl 4: S164–S192.

Bolanowski M, Nilsson BE. Assessment of human body composition using dual-energy x-ray absorptiometry and bioelectrical impedance analysis. *Med Sci Monit.* Sep–Oct 2001;7(5):1029–1033.

Deurenberg P, Deurenberg-Yap M, Guricci S. Asians are different from Caucasians and from each other in their body mass index/body fat percent relationship. *Obes Rev.* Aug 2002;3(3):141–146.

Ellis KJ. Selected body composition methods can be used in field studies. *J Nutr.* May 2001;131(5):1589S–1595S.

Flegal KM, Wei R, Ogden CL, Freedman DS, Johnson CL, Curtin LR. Characterizing extreme values of body mass index-for-age by using the 2000 Centers for Disease Control and Prevention growth charts. *Am J Clin Nutr.* Nov 2009;90(5):1314–1320.

Flodmark CE, Lissau I, Moreno LA, Pietrobelli A, Widhalm K. New insights into the field of children and adolescents' obesity: the European perspective. *Int J Obes Relat Metab Disord.* Oct 2004;28(10): 1189–1196.

Hubbard VS. Defining overweight and obesity: what are the issues? *Am J Clin Nutr.* Nov 2000;72(5):1067–1068.

Lee SY, Gallagher D. Assessment methods in human body composition. *Curr Opin Clin Nutr Metab Care.* Sep 2008;11(5):566–572.

NHLBI. National Heart, Lung, and Blood Institute. Clinical guidelines on the identification, evaluation, and treatment of overweight and obesity in adults: executive summary. Vol. No. 98–4083. Bethesda, MD: National Institutes of Health; 1998.

Poirier P. Recurrent cardiovascular events in contemporary cardiology: obesity patients should not rest in PEACE. *Eur Heart J.* Jun 2006;27(12): 1390–1391.

Sturm R. Increases in morbid obesity in the USA: 2000–2005. *Public Health.* Jul 2007;121(7):492–496.

Wang J, Thornton JC, Kolesnik S, Pierson RN, Jr. Anthropometry in body composition. An overview. *Ann N Y Acad Sci.* May 2000;904:317–326.

WHO. World Health Organization. Appropriate body-mass index for Asian populations and its implications for policy and intervention strategies. *Lancet.* Jan 10 2004;363(9403):157–163.

CHAPTER 3

CAUSES OF OBESITY

READER OBJECTIVES

- Describe how individual biologic factors influence obesity
- Explain how energy balance is related to obesity
- Indentify components that contribute to metabolic rate and their implications for obesity management
- Discuss factors that have an impact on basal metabolic rate variability
- Describe methods of measurement or estimation of energy expenditure
- Compute resting metabolic rate using equations
- Summarize research regarding trends that contribute to increased energy intake in the United States
- Compare biologic and endocrinologic mediators (e.g., leptin, ghrelin, neurotransmitters) that regulate energy balance
- Discuss implications of gene, environment, and behavior interactions on obesity

CHAPTER OUTLINE

Factors That Contribute to Obesity

Why are Americans overweight? Is it fast food? Supersized portions? Too much time in front of the TV? Experts have proposed various explanations for overweight and obesity. However, the answer is not clear cut. Individual variation in body fat storage is based on a complex interplay of genetic, biologic, behavioral, and environmental factors. Obesity is fundamentally caused by an imbalance between food and activity: too much energy in and too little energy out. The degree of imbalance is influenced by how an individual's food intake and physical activity are affected by biologic and environmental factors. As a consequence of modern lifestyle and environment, we now have access to large amounts of palatable, high-calorie food and a limited need for physical activity. Humans evolved in an environment that required vigorous physical work, and it was characterized by cycles of feast and famine. To survive, humans developed an innate preference for sweet, high-fat, high-calorie foods that could increase body fat stores that could be drawn upon during times when food was scarce. These natural defenses against starvation are counterproductive in our current environment where food is easily and consistently accessible and technology has reduced the requirement for daily physical work. **Figure 3.1**

shows that environmental, behavioral, genetic and metabolic factors all contribute to energy balance.

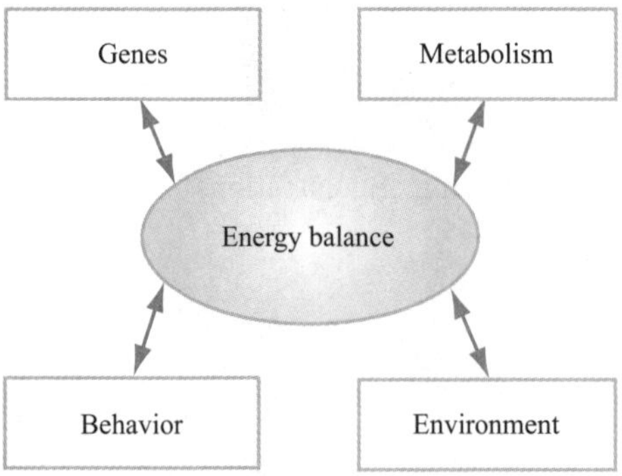

Energy Balance

To understand obesity, we must understand the components of energy balance and the metabolic and genetic elements that govern them. The balance between energy intake from food and energy expenditure determines how much energy is available to be stored in periods of energy abundance and how it is released in times of energy shortage. Body fat storage is based on the first law of thermodynamics, the principle of conservation of energy. The law states that energy may be changed

FIGURE **3.1**   **Factors that affect energy balance.**

BOX 3.1   Definition of *Calorie*

A calorie* is a measure of energy. It is defined as the amount of energy (in the form of heat) it takes to raise 1 g of water 1°C. Food components provide varying amounts of energy. The units are generally reported as kilocalorie per gram (kcal/g).

> Protein = 4 kcal/g
> Fat = 9 kcal/g
> Carbohydrate = 4 kcal/g
> Alcohol = 7 kcal/g

The excess energy consumed from any of these components can be stored in the form of body fat. Each pound of body fat represents approximately 3,500 kcal of stored energy.

---

*In the general description of energy intake, the word *calorie* is often used instead of the more precise scientific term *kilocalorie* (*kcal*), which is equal to 1,000 calories of energy. The term *kcal* is used most often with numbers or measurements. For instance, calories listed on food labels are kcal. Throughout this text the terms *calorie* and *kilocalorie* are interchangeable.

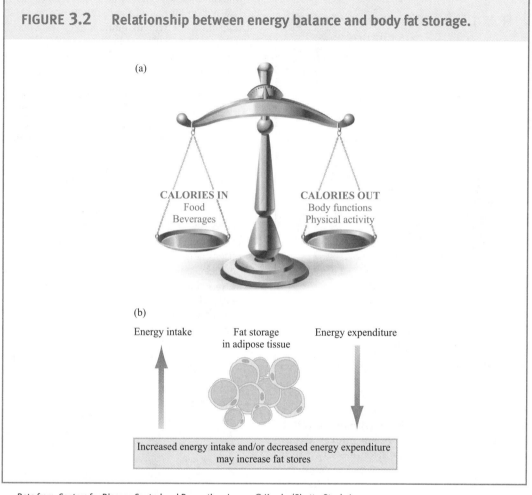

FIGURE 3.2   Relationship between energy balance and body fat storage.

(a)

CALORIES IN
Food
Beverages

CALORIES OUT
Body functions
Physical activity

(b)

Energy intake   Fat storage   Energy expenditure
in adipose tissue

Increased energy intake and/or decreased energy expenditure
may increase fat stores

Data from: Centers for Disease Control and Prevention. *Image*: © Kraska/ShutterStock, Inc.

from one form to another, but cannot be created or destroyed. Energy obtained from food must be used for essential metabolic processes, muscular work, heat production, or storage. **Figure 3.2** shows how energy intake must be used or stored—it does not merely disappear.

Stable energy balance occurs when calories taken in are equal to the calories expended, and body weight is maintained. Positive energy balance happens when the calories consumed are greater than the calories expended. Weight is gained and fat stores are increased. In negative energy balance, energy consumed is less than energy expended.

Body fat stores can be mobilized to make up the caloric deficiency and in this way body fat stores are reduced.

Metabolic Rate

Metabolism refers to all of the chemical reactions that direct normal body functioning and go on continuously inside the body. These processes require energy from food. The speed at which food energy is used in the body is the *metabolic rate*. As shown in **Figure 3.3** energy expenditure can be divided into three main components: basal

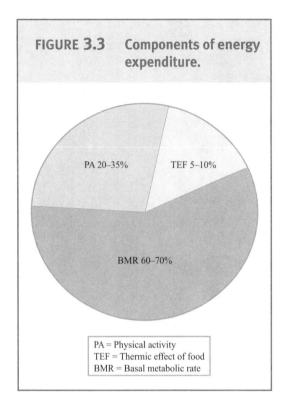

FIGURE **3.3** **Components of energy expenditure.**

PA 20–35%

TEF 5–10%

BMR 60–70%

PA = Physical activity
TEF = Thermic effect of food
BMR = Basal metabolic rate

metabolic rate, physical activity, and thermic effect of food (Lowell, 2000). **Basal metabolic rate (BMR)** is also called **basal energy expenditure (BEE)** and it accounts for about two-thirds of daily calorie expenditure. It is the amount of energy expended each day to maintain the basic functions such as heartbeat, respiration, and body temperature. This would be equal to the energy required just to rest in bed all day. BMR for most adults is between 1,200 and 1,800 kcal per day. Energy used during movement and physical activity in a normally active person requires about 20 percent of daily energy expenditure. The thermic effect of food, or the energy required to eat, digest, and metabolize food, is about 10 percent of total daily energy use.

BMR varies among individuals, and a key determinant of the variation is the individual's proportion of lean muscle mass. Reduction in lean muscle mass reduces BMR. Muscle is metabolically more active than fat cells and it requires more calories for work and maintenance. Because the

BMR accounts for the largest portion of daily energy expenditure, it is important to preserve muscle mass for weight management (Ravussin, 1992). Variability in BMR among apparently similar individuals can be influenced by numerous other factors including:

- Age: BMR slows with age, due to a loss in muscle tissue as well as hormonal changes.
- Body size: Larger bodies have larger muscle mass and organ tissues that require a higher BMR.
- Dieting, fasting, or starvation: When too few calories are available, metabolism slows to conserve energy. A loss of lean muscle tissue further contributes to a drop in BMR.
- Emotions or stress: Increased counter-regulatory hormones can influence how quickly the body uses energy.
- Genetic predisposition: Many of these factors are influenced by some degree of genetic control.
- Growth: There is a higher energy demand per unit of body weight in growing infants, children, and adolescents.
- Infection or illness: BMR increases to mount an immune response and to repair or replace damaged tissues.
- Medications: Drugs that are central nervous system stimulants may increase BMR.
- Sex: In general, men have a faster metabolism than women because they tend to have a higher proportion of lean body tissue.
- Temperature: In response to cool temperatures extra energy is used to produce more body heat. In hot conditions increased energy is needed to maintain normal body temperature by increased perspiring and respiration.
- Time of day: Energy expenditure is continuous, but the rate varies throughout the day. The lowest rate of energy expenditure is usually in the early morning.

It has also been shown that some constituents of the diet, including caffeine in tea and coffee, alcohol, and even spices such as chili pepper, horseradish, and mustard, could increase metabolic rate (Henry, 1986; Westerterp, 2004).

Although these factors affect metabolism in general, BMR itself is not easy to change. The best opportunities to prevent or reduce fat storage are alterations in the other contributors to energy balance: food consumption and activity level.

Energy Expenditure Terminology, Measurement, and Equations

The most accurate methods to determine basal energy expenditure use **direct calorimetry**, a measure of heat released from a person's body (or **thermogenesis**) and measurements of exhaled gas exchange in participants who occupy a metabolic chamber.

Because BMR assessment with a metabolic chamber is not generally practical, an alternative method of estimating energy expenditure may be applied. Researchers and clinicians use **indirect calorimetry** to measure **resting metabolic rate (RMR)** or **resting energy expenditure (REE)**. RMR evaluation requires only that the individual be fasting and resting for about 30 minutes. Metabolic carts are computerized portable instruments used in this indirect measure of RMR. The amount of inspired and expired air is determined with a mask that covers the nose and mouth. Specific equations are used to calculate total energy expenditure from the difference in volume of oxygen inhaled and carbon dioxide exhaled. Health professionals may also assess RMR indirectly using a small, hand-held device. Subjects hold the unit while breathing through an attached mouthpiece or face mask and sensors measure oxygen consumption that is converted to a digital readout of RMR in kcal/day.

There is a close correlation between BMR and body fat storage. A low BMR is a risk factor for weight gain (Daniels, 2005). The American Dietetic Association (ADA) adult weight management guidelines promote the idea that a resting energy expenditure measurement should be part of a complete dietary assessment (Seagle, 2009). Because RMR measurement with either direct or indirect

BOX 3.2 Metabolic Chamber

A metabolic chamber is a room with highly controlled conditions where metabolic testing takes place while the subject eats, sleeps, and performs various physical activities. To measure BMR, subjects must spend the night sleeping in the facility so that tests can take place as soon as the person awakes. The BMR protocol may require 8 hours of sleep, 12 hours of fasting, and the subject in a reclining position in a darkened room at a temperature of 26–30°C.

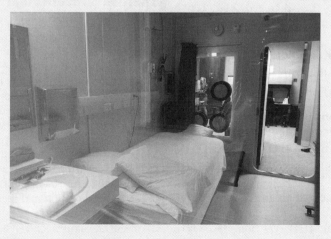

Photograph: © T. Ortega Gaines/MCT/Landov.

calorimetry is expensive and time-consuming and not always available in clinical practice, alternative estimates of BMR can be made with various predictive equations. Two examples of calculations used to estimate metabolic rate are the Harris-Benedict and the Mifflin-St Jeor equations. These equations are sex-specific and take height, weight, and age into account. The Harris-Benedict equations for basal energy expenditure developed in 1919 to establish normal standards are still widely used today for clinical and research purposes. While they appear valid, there is evidence that the Harris-Benedict equations may overestimate BMR in obese persons (Frankenfield, 2003). Because average adult body weight and activity levels are different than they were in the early 20th century, the Mifflin-St Jeor equations were proposed as more contemporary alternatives to the Harris-Benedict equations (Mifflin, 1990). Recent studies report that both prediction equations may be equally useful for population or group assessment, but each has wide variations for individuals when compared with indirect calorimetry (Amirkalali, 2008).

Equations for Calculation of BMR

Where:

W = weight in kilograms

H = height in centimeters

A = age

The Harris-Benedict equation for BMR:

For men: $(13.75 \times W) + (5 \times H) - (6.76 \times A) + 66$

For women: $(9.56 \times W) + (1.85 \times H) - (4.68 \times A) + 655$

The Mifflin-St Jeor equation for BMR:

For men: $(10 \times W) + (6.25 \times H) - (5 \times A) + 5$

For women: $(10 \times W) + (6.25 \times H) - (5 \times A) - 161$

Sample calculations using the Harris-Benedict equation (rounded values):

Man: 21 years old, 5 ft 10 in. (171 cm), 155 lb (70 kg)

$66.5 + [13.8 \times (70 \text{ kg})] + [5 \times (171 \text{ cm})] - [6.8 \times (21)]$
$= 1,745$ kcal/day

Woman: 21 years old, 5 ft 10 in. (171 cm), 155 lb (70 kg)

$655.1 + [9.6 \times (70 \text{ kg})] + [1.8 \times (171 \text{ cm})] - [4.7 \times (21)]$
$= 1,536$ kcal/day

Because the largest contributor to variation in individual BMR is the ratio of lean to fat body mass, a disadvantage of these equations is that they do not take body composition into account. A person with an above average amount of muscle will have a higher BMR than calculated, and the daily calorie needs estimated by equation will be too low for weight maintenance. A person with a below average amount of muscle or excess fat will have a lower metabolic rate than computed, and the suggested daily calories will be too high. Details about how these and other equations can be applied to obese clients can be found in the article by David Frankenfield and colleagues listed in the References section.

As BMR and RMR represent only resting energy expenditure, to estimate the required calories for daily living the BMR calculation must be multiplied by an appropriate activity factor (McArdle, 1996). The resulting number is the recommended daily calorie intake to maintain current body weight. Activity factors give a general estimate of energy expended. There are various opinions of what the factors should be when considering individual differences in intensity of physical activity. One categorization scheme is shown in **Table 3.1**. Online calculators include activity factors to make it easy to determine daily calorie requirements. Websites for these calculators are listed in the Resources section of this chapter.

Thermic Effect of Food

Because an increase in oxygen consumption and basal energy expenditure is needed to digest and metabolize food, BMR rises after eating. This rise in metabolic rate is termed the **thermic effect of food (TEF)** (Rothwell, 1981). The increase occurs shortly after eating and peaks 2 to 3 hours later. On average, TEF requires about 10% of total calories consumed. However, TEF varies depending on the size of the meal and the types of nutrients and foods consumed. Studies on the thermic effect of food show that the body uses carbohydrates efficiently so that 5 to 10% of calories in carbohydrates are used for digestion and metabolism. Fat is the most economical source of energy; it requires 0 to 3% of the fat calories for transfer, metabolism, and storage. In contrast, about 20 to 30% of the calories

TABLE 3.1 Activity Factors for Daily Calorie Requirements Calculations

Activity factor	Category	Definition
1.2	Sedentary	Little or no exercise and desk job.
1.375	Lightly active	Light exercise or sports 1–3 days a week or walking 2 hours per day.
1.55	Moderately active	Moderate exercise or sports 3–5 days a week or walking 3 hours per day.
1.725	Very active	Hard exercise or sports 6–7 days a week or walking 4 hours per day.
1.9	Extremely active	Hard daily exercise or sports and physical job that includes walking 5 or more hours per day.

Adapted from: McArdle WD, Katch FI, Katch VL, eds. *Exercise Physiology: Energy, Nutrition, and Human Performance.* 4th ed. Baltimore, MD: Williams & Wilkins; 1996.

in protein are used for its digestion and metabolism (Halton, 2004). The high thermic expenditure of protein may be due to the fact that dietary protein metabolism requires energy to synthesize body proteins and to produce urea for excretion of nitrogen by-products (Robinson, 1990).

BOX 3.3 Thermic Effect of Foods

- Fats raise BMR about 4%
- Carbohydrates raise BMR about 6%
- Proteins raise BMR up to 30%

Energy Used During Physical Activity

The direct effects of physical activity interventions on energy expenditure are relatively small when placed in the context of total daily energy demands. Although energy expenditure for physical activity is highly variable, in a normally active person it may account for 20 percent of daily energy use while the BMR requires as much as two-thirds of daily energy intake. However, physical activity does have an important influence on BMR and body weight maintenance. When daily activity is sufficient to sustain lean muscle mass, BMR also will be maintained or increased.

Environmental Contributors to Increased Energy Intake

Increasingly, the health environment in the United States has become **obesogenic**—a term used to describe the worldwide economic and cultural changes that have altered food selection and physical activity in ways that promote weight gain. Though these conditions vary greatly by region, there are some common trends. As incomes rise and populations become more urban, traditional diets high in complex carbohydrates are replaced with more fats and sugars. At the same time, less physically demanding work is required due to the increasing use of labor-saving technology in the home and at work. There is easy access to a wide variety of good-tasting, inexpensive, calorie-rich foods that are served and marketed in large portions. Fast food outlets provide a tempting combination of convenience and large portions at low cost. As a result, we eat more food than ever before (Variyam 2005). On the energy output side, many Americans lead essentially sedentary lives. People sit all day at computers and use cars to get to and from work. Even leisure time is spent in sedentary activities such as watching television, shopping, and communicating or playing games on computers.

A Nation at Risk: Obesity in America, published by the Robert Wood Johnson Foundation in 2005, reviewed scientific research studies concerning changes in the eating patterns of Americans over several decades. The report cited three major food trends that contribute to obesity (AHA, 2005):

1. More food and beverage calories are conveniently available.
2. Bigger portion sizes are accepted and expected.
3. A major increase in eating away from home.

Food Availability

The USDA Economic Research Service (ERS) Food Availability Data System reports suggest that food availability in all major food groups has consistently increased over recent decades. As the food supply grows, each person has the opportunity to consume more energy, or calories. In the early 1980s, there was enough food available in the marketplaces to provide an average of 3,300 calories per capita per day. National farm policy changed and farmers were encouraged to grow more food. The result was that American farmers produce enough food to furnish every person with about 3,900 calories a day. Due to increased supply, food prices in stores and restaurants have declined relative to prices of other goods and in relation to income. Between 1952 and 2003, the ratio of food prices to the prices of all other goods fell by 12%. The average family spent just 9.9% of their income on food in 2006 compared with 14.8% in the 1960s (ERS, 2012). Advances in food processing and packaging are instrumental in encouraging Americans to consume these extra, low-cost calories as a multitude of ready-to-eat foods are now readily available (Variyam 2005). It is interesting to look back even further in time at the tables created by the ERS that display the proportion of an individual's disposable personal income spent on food since 1929. There is a website for the tables listed in the Resources section of this chapter.

A 2010 study assessed the availability and accessibility of energy-dense snack foods and beverages that have been implicated as contributors to obesity. Observations of 1,082 retail stores in 19 US cities determined that snack food was widely available in retail stores whose primary business is not food. There were snack foods in 96% of pharmacies, 94% of gasoline stations, 22% of furniture stores, and 16% of apparel stores. The authors concluded that the ubiquity of these products makes it easy to consume excess energy (Farley, 2010).

Another factor that contributes to easy food availability is that food preparation does not have to take much time. In 1965 it took a housewife more than 2 hours per day to shop, cook, and clean up from meals. Meal preparation took half that time in 1995. Researchers have suggested that the increase in food consumption permitted by the falling time cost of preparing and acquiring food is a major cause behind the surge in obesity since 1980 (Variyam, 2005).

Beverages Add More Calories

Sugar-sweetened beverages, including sweetened fruit drinks, carbonated drinks, and sports beverages account for nearly half the added sugars in the US diet (Guthrie, 2000). Millions of vending machines dispense billions of soft drinks. In the past, soft drinks were sold in 6-oz bottles. Then they increased to 12-oz cans. Now the soft drink trend is toward serving sizes of 20 oz or more. Most individuals will drink the entire contents of a can or bottle, particularly when they assume that the container is a single serving (Johnson, 2007). Sugar-sweetened drinks can contribute to overweight and obesity because they provide large amounts of liquid calories that may not be recognized by appetite feedback mechanisms. People normally respond to increased energy intake by eating less after consuming a large meal. That adjustment occurs more readily with solid foods than with beverages. Lack of compensation for liquid calorie intake was seen in a study of men and women who were given 450 extra calories per day as either three 12-oz cans of soda or 45 large jelly beans. Participants who ate the candy ate less at a later meal and adjusted for the extra energy while those who got the liquid calories made no compensation and their daily energy intake increased. The study researcher stated, "Liquid calories don't trip our satiety mechanisms. They just don't register" (DiMeglio, 2000). Multiple studies indicate a consistent association between sweetened drink consumption and increased energy intake. It is remarkable that a single food source can have such a substantial impact on total energy intake and increased risk for obesity (Vartanian, 2007).

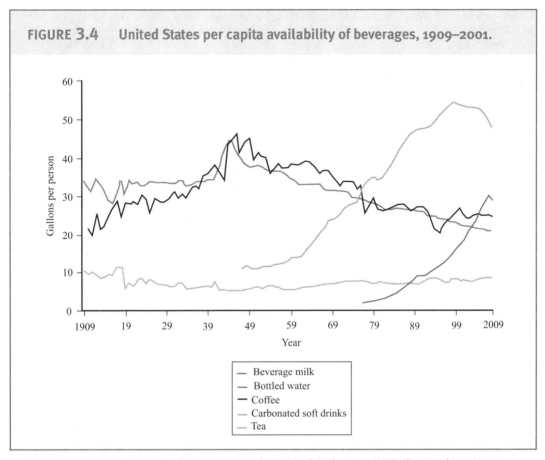

FIGURE **3.4**   United States per capita availability of beverages, 1909–2001.

Beverage milk
Bottled water
Coffee
Carbonated soft drinks
Tea

Source: Economic Research Service (ERS), U.S. Department of Agriculture (USDA). Food Availability (Per Capita) Data System. http://www.ers.usda.gov/Data/FoodConsumption/app/reports/displayCommodities.aspx?reportName=Beverages%20by%20 individual%20beverage&id=42#startForm.

Figure 3.4 shows the trends in consumption of beverages over the last century.

Increased Portion Sizes

Wherever Americans purchase or consume food, increasingly larger servings are represented as a single portion. The maximum serving size of fries sold at McDonald's has increased from 210 calories in 1955 to 610 calories for a supersized portion today. In the 1950s, the standard size bottle of Coca Cola was about 6 oz. Many convenience stores in the United States commonly sell 64-oz soft drinks (2 qt). Muffins, cookies, and candy are also

available in larger and larger sizes that provide 500 calories or more in each apparently single-serving package. To show how portions today compare with portion sizes 20 years ago the National Institutes of Health has an interactive website called "Portion Distortion" (see the Resources section in this chapter).

Eating Away from Home

The relative decline in the cost of food means that more people can afford the convenience of eating out and purchasing food away from home. In 1966, only 24% of all food expenses went toward food prepared away from home. By 2009, the percentage nearly doubled to 49% (ERS, 2012). Meals eaten away from home permit access to large quantities of calorie-rich foods. As the foodservice industry offers more choices, from fast food to a wide array of ethnic restaurants, dining out provides convenience and variety. All those meals have contributed to the increase in overweight and obesity as there is evidence that foods eaten away from home are more calorie-dense (provide more calories per serving) than foods prepared at home (McCrory, 1999).

Impact of Socioeconomic Status

Socioeconomic status (SES) is associated with body weight in the United States. The highest obesity rates are linked to low-income, low-education, minority status, and a higher incidence of poverty (Lantz, 1998; CDC, 2011). Important economic factors that have a significant effect on weight and health are inequitable access to healthy foods and a safe environment for physical activity. Researchers have shown that low-income neighborhoods attract more fast food outlets and convenience stores as opposed to full-service supermarkets and grocery stores. Every day, one out of four Americans eats fast food and a 2004 study revealed that 30% of children eat fast food on a daily basis (Bowman, 2004). Most people choose these food outlets for the convenience, and lack of time leads many people to the drive through. Obviously this provides easy energy access without much physical energy expended. Economics plays a part as well as fast food restaurants are often the cheapest option. Because prepared and packaged foods made with refined flours and inexpensive fats and sugars cost less than whole grains, fruits, and vegetables, it is more difficult for people with low income to select the foods that are associated with a healthful weight control diet. By contrast, more affluent people generally have access to stores with a variety of nutritious foods and fresher produce as well as convenient opportunities for physical activity (Drewnowski, 2009).

Reduced Opportunity for Physical Activity

Along with a growing tendency to consume more calories, Americans have become less active compared with previous decades. Given a technology-driven workforce that has shifted from physically demanding labor to sedentary occupations, a daily job for most people no longer provides opportunity for physical activity. In addition, the number of hours employees work each week has been increasing and so there is even less possibility for physical activity during leisure time (Hu, 2001).

Metabolic and Genetic Contributions to Eating Behavior

For most dieters weight loss is not permanent. Weight regain was once thought to be the result of inadequate changes to diet and exercise programs or lack of knowledge or willpower. Now, experts believe that the explanation is not that straightforward. Although eating is generally believed to be a voluntary, conscious behavior, evidence suggests that energy intake and physical expenditure are controlled by involuntary biologic systems (Friedman, 2009). These complex pathways involve fat cells, hormones, and neurochemicals in the brain that regulate the balance between energy input and energy expenditure. An outcome of human evolution is a metabolism that favors energy storage. Calorie reduction may bring about short-term weight decrease but long-term maintenance of weight loss is difficult due to the regulatory mechanisms that preserve accumulated body fat. Defense against loss of energy stores assures that deviations in levels of adiposity are countered with compensatory changes in appetite and energy expenditure that maintain body fat levels. Because these physiologic mechanisms protect against starvation by causing an increase in appetite and a decrease in energy expenditure, it is very difficult to keep off the weight that is intentionally reduced (Cummings, 2003; Glandt, 2011).

It is evident that eating is a behavior that merges input from the external physical environment with internal physiologic processes. Two biologic pathways, the **homeostatic** system and the **hedonic** system, link the physiologic, behavioral, and environmental influences on food intake (Blundell, 2006).

Homeostatic Controls

Energy balance and fat storage are homeostatic processes, in which the hypothalamus area of the brain is a central controller of food intake. The hypothalamus receives and transmits information about hunger and satiety, monitors nutrient status signals from the digestive tract and fat cells, and integrates this information to direct food intake and energy expenditure. The signaling is centered in the arcuate nucleus, a group of cells in the hypothalamus. Neurons in the arcuate nucleus express the neuropeptide proopiomelanocortin (POMC), which inhibits appetite, and neuropeptide Y (NPY), which increases appetite (Morton, 2006). These neurochemicals protect against weight gain as well as weight loss, at least in normal-weight individuals (Zheng, 2008). When the effect of these neurons is balanced, body fat storage is stable.

Homeostatic regulation of energy intake involves short-term signals that control hunger, food intake, and satiety, and long-term signals that defend energy stores and maintain lean tissue. In short-term regulation, messages from the stomach and intestine give the brain information about current energy intake while long-term signals inform the brain of changes in body fat mass (Woods, 2004). One such signal that causes eating cessation is distention of the stomach and upper intestine. In addition to the nerves that sense these physical changes, several intestinal hormones alert the brain that the stomach is getting full. The absence as well as the presence of nutrients in the gastrointestinal tract inform the brain about hunger and satiety and signal when to stop or start eating. As opposed to hormones and mechanisms that stop or slow eating, the hormone ghrelin is secreted from the mucosa of an empty stomach, stimulates appetite, and promotes food intake. It increases shortly before eating and decreases rapidly with food consumption (Cummings, 2001). Ghrelin is often called the hunger hormone because it is produced in response to meal schedules or even the sight or smell of food and it is thought to be responsible for the feeling recognized as hunger. Appetite-stimulating ghrelin levels are also increased in response to negative energy balance, such as with fasting or weight loss (Hansen, 2002).

Compared with lean individuals, ghrelin may act differently in obese people. Baseline circulating ghrelin levels are lower with obesity, and the normal **postprandial** (following a meal) decline in ghrelin levels does not occur, which can lead to unregulated appetite and weight gain (Chan, 2004).

Long-term signals about energy storage come from fat cells. Fat cells, also termed **adipocytes**, are not just inert energy storage organs that accumulate and release fatty acids ingested from food. They also secrete a wide array of biologically active molecules including the hormone leptin (Bray, 2005). Leptin (from the Greek *leptos*, meaning thin or lean) acts as a fat regulator. With increased body fat, adipose tissue secretes higher levels of leptin. As the amount of fat stored in adipocytes rises, more leptin is released into the blood as a signal to the brain that the body has enough energy stores. The hormone binds to leptin receptors in the brain, including the hypothalamus where it inhibits NPY receptors and stimulates POMC receptors. The result is a feeling of satiety, reduced food intake, and increased energy expenditure. On the other hand, when body fat is reduced, leptin levels are also reduced. When this happens, the hypothalamus detects a decrease in fat stores and it triggers an increase in food intake to replenish the fat in the cells. **Figure 3.5** illustrates how leptin levels support a relatively constant weight over time (Friedman, 1998).

Leptin was discovered in the 1990s in obese mice that carried a gene that made them unable to produce any leptin. When absolute leptin deficiency exists in mice and humans it causes severe obesity. The discovery of the fat-regulating hormone leptin was met with the enthusiastic expectation that injecting obese patients with leptin could produce weight loss. Unfortunately, clinical trials of obese participants conducted in 1999 showed that, even when they were given high doses of leptin, they lost only a small amount of weight. Although there are millions of obese people in the world, absolute leptin deficiency is extremely rare in humans (Bray, 2004). After years of study, researchers have found only a few dozen individuals who have a congenital leptin deficit and a high degree of obesity. When these individuals are given supplemental injections, they lose weight. Most people with obesity have very high levels of leptin in their bloodstreams related to high levels of body fat. Rather than possessing a leptin deficiency, obese individuals are likely to be insensitive to the effects

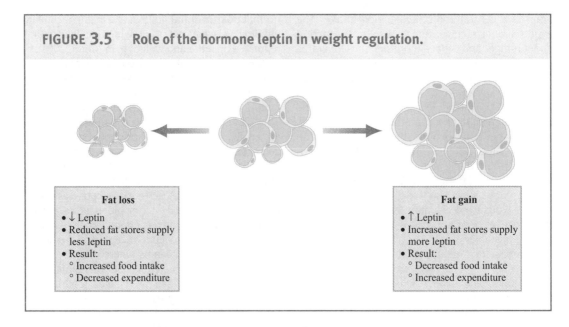

FIGURE **3.5**   Role of the hormone leptin in weight regulation.

Fat loss
- ↓ Leptin
- Reduced fat stores supply less leptin
- Result:
  ◦ Increased food intake
  ◦ Decreased expenditure

Fat gain
- ↑ Leptin
- Increased fat stores supply more leptin
- Result:
  ◦ Decreased food intake
  ◦ Increased expenditure

of the hormone, and injecting more leptin is of no benefit (Heymsfield, 1999).

Hedonic System

Research studies of the effects of leptin and neuropeptides on homeostatic control of food intake focus on the "metabolic brain" (Zheng, 2008). Functional appetite control is also driven by environmental and social cues that stimulate the hedonic system (Blundell, 2004). Humans choose to eat simply for enjoyment or companionship without regard for physiologic needs. The role of the "cognitive and emotional brain" must be considered to appreciate how metabolic need is translated into behavior that guides daily food choices. The hedonic system is less well studied than the homeostatic physiology and the interactions of the two systems are not well defined (Zheng, 2008). Hedonic control of eating is centered in the **cortico-limbic** network. With the aid of cognitive, visual, and olfactory cues, this network of nerves and hormones responds to the emotional aspects of food. Overweight and obesity could result when aspects of food consumption such as the stimulation and pleasure of eating, delicious taste, and desirability override those homeostatic controls that prevent overconsumption. The high fat and

sugar content of highly palatable foods may alter homeostatic appetite control (Seagle, 2009).

Genetic Contributions to Obesity

Lifestyle choices may be voluntary but there is also the underlying command from genetic sources. It is estimated that genetics accounts for about 30 to 40% of the differences in weight among individuals (Wajchenberg, 2000). Studies of twins and adopted children demonstrate that there is greater body weight similarity among monozygotic (identical) twins compared to dizygotic (fraternal) twins. A study of adult male identical twins shows the impact of genetics on weight gain. Twin pairs were fed an extra 1,000 kcal per day. There were large differences among the various twin pairs as weight gain among all the participants ranged from about 10 to 30 lb. Some twin pairs gained much more weight than other pairs. However, the concordance, or the similarity, within pairs was strongly significant for body weight and measures of fat distribution (Bouchard, 1990). Further evidence of genetic influence is demonstrated in a study of 540 adult adoptees as the adoptees' weight was strongly related to the BMI of their biologic parents, but it was not significantly related to the BMI of their adoptive parents (Stunkard, 1986).

BOX 3.4 Risk of Childhood Obesity Is Closely Tied to a Parent's Obesity

---

A child's chance of becoming obese is:

7% with no obese parents

40% with one obese parent

80% with two obese parents

Data from: Nguyen VT, Larson DE, Johnson RK, Goran MI. Fat intake and adiposity in children of lean and obese parents. *Am J Clin Nutr*. Apr 1996; 63(4):507–513.

While the role of genetic determinants of obesity is intriguing, it cannot explain the recent epidemic of obesity. Our human genome has not drastically changed in just a few decades. Furthermore, not all individuals exposed to an abundant food supply become obese, and not all obese people develop adverse health consequences. This diversity in how people respond to the same environmental conditions suggest that, while genes do play an important role in energy balance, genes themselves do not determine whether a person is obese or thin. They regulate individual susceptibility to weight gain in response to environmental factors. Although genes influence susceptibility, the occurrence of obesity depends on an individual's ability to ignore the environmental cues that encourage excess food consumption and discourage physical activity. This is not an easy task considering daily exposure to obesogenic factors that include (Cohen-Cole, 2008):

- A wide variety of inexpensive and easily accessible food is available around the clock.
- Food can be purchased at school, work, and play.
- People can buy food without getting out of a car and can eat while driving.
- Cultural cues encourage excesses of consumption because food plays a central role in community and family functions.

- There may be an expectation that appreciation and gratitude are shown by eating large amounts of specially prepared food.

Although the human genome has not changed significantly from the time of hunter-gathers, our environment has been fundamentally transformed. Humans evolved in an environment that required high energy to obtain an adequate amount of food (Booth, 2002). It is postulated that early humans were exposed to two basic food environments: one of plenty and one of scarcity. In an environment where food was plentiful and consistently available, there was no critical need for genes that directed increased adipose tissue storage. On the other hand, people who lived in an environment where food was scarce inherited a "thrifty" gene system because they needed to be able to survive on a small amount of food and readily store extra energy for future use (Ravussin, 1990). Those who could store energy in times of plenty were more likely to survive periods of famine and this tendency was passed to their offspring. An environment in which food is plentiful now challenges the same thrifty genes that made it easier for early humans to survive occasional lack of food. A dramatic example of how the gene-environment hypothesis can be applied is the variation in BMI among Pima Indians. Pima who moved from Mexico to live in Arizona have a very high incidence of obesity, while those living in rural Mexico do not. A survey showed the average BMI was 24.9 for Pimas who lived in Mexico and 33.4 for those living in Arizona. The difference is attributed to a high-fat, calorie-dense diet and sedentary lifestyle adopted by the tribe living the United States, while the Mexican tribe members follow a more traditional low-fat diet and have a high activity level (Schulz, 2006).

Summary

There is no way around the fact that obesity occurs when there is a positive energy balance. Unwanted or unintentional fat storage is due to a discrepancy between the levels of energy intake and energy expenditure that are intentionally controlled, and the levels of energy expenditure that are involuntary, such as those that comprise the BMR. Contributing to increased fat storage is an environment where an abundance of food is easily accessible without need for much physical activity. Excess energy storage, now considered to be a health problem, was probably advantageous when food was less available and high amounts of physical activity were a way of life. Although genetically programmed physiologic controls may influence eating and physical activity behaviors and susceptibility to store fat, they are not solely responsible for whether a person become obese. Humans make conscious, voluntary decisions and choices even if they are shaped by a subconscious component. The critical question to manage the obesity crisis is, what individual and population efforts can help to achieve a healthful energy balance within the context of these biologic, genetic, and behavioral factors?

Critical Thinking Questions

Question: What factors in your daily life allow food to be convenient and quickly available?

Question: We live in an environment where there is easy accessibility to food that is tasty and cheap, and you can eat it with one hand. Health experts have argued that, given that situation, the current focus on changing dietary components or behavior is most likely to be futile. What is your opinion?

Question: How does leptin help to regulate to body fat storage? What are the physiologic and behavioral responses when fat stores decrease? What are the responses when fat stores increase?

Question: Considering energy balance, discuss the importance of the fact that homeostatic and hedonic systems do not appear to be integrated relative to obesity.

Question: Why is an obesogenic lifestyle or environment probably a necessary but insufficient factor to increase the risk of obesity?

Resources

Nutritional Calculator

http://www.workoutsforwomen.com/nutritional_calculator.asp

Adult Energy Needs and BMI Calculator

http://www.bcm.edu/cnrc/caloriesneed.htm

Portion Distortion! Do You Know How Food Portions Have Changed in 20 Years?

http://hp2010.nhlbihin.net/portion/

Economic Research Service (ERS), United States Department of Agriculture (USDA), Food Availability (Per Capita) Data System

http://www.ers.usda.gov/Data/FoodConsumption

ERS has been calculating the amount of food commodities available for consumption for decades. Users can download spreadsheets from all three data series or use the custom query feature to get tables or charts for specific food groups, individual commodities, and years.

USDA-ERS Food CPI and Expenditures: Food Expenditure Tables, Table 7
http://www.ers.usda.gov/Briefing/CPIFoodAndExpenditures/Data/Expenditures_tables/
This site shows food expenditures by families and individuals as a share of disposable personal income.
United States Department of Agriculture Economic Research Service Table 97—Percent of Household Final Consumption Expenditures Spent on Food, Alcoholic Beverages, and Tobacco That Were Consumed at Home, by Selected Countries, 2009
http://www.ers.usda.gov/Briefing/CPIFoodAndExpenditures/

References

AHA. *A Nation at Risk: Obesity in the United States, a Statistical Sourcebook of Facts About Obesity.* Dallas, TX: American Heart Association and the Robert Wood Johnson Foundation; 2005.

Amirkalali B, Hosseini S, Heshmat R, Larijani B. Comparison of Harris Benedict and Mifflin-St Jeor equations with indirect calorimetry in evaluating resting energy expenditure. *Indian J Med Sci.* Jul 2008;62(7): 283–290.

Blundell JE. Perspective on the central control of appetite. *Obesity (Silver Spring).* Jul 2006;14 Suppl 4: 160S–163S.

Blundell JE, Finlayson G. Is susceptibility to weight gain characterized by homeostatic or hedonic risk factors for overconsumption? *Physiol Behav.* Aug 2004; 82(1):21–25.

Booth FW, Chakravarthy MV, Spangenburg EE. Exercise and gene expression: physiological regulation of the human genome through physical activity. *J Physiol.* Sep 1 2002;543(Pt 2):399–411.

Bouchard C, Tremblay A, Despres JP, et al. The response to long-term overfeeding in identical twins. *N Engl J Med.* May 24 1990;322(21):1477–1482.

Bowman SA, Vinyard BT. Fast food consumption of U.S. adults: impact on energy and nutrient intakes and overweight status. *J Am Coll Nutr.* Apr 2004;23(2): 163–168.

Bray GA. Obesity is a chronic, relapsing neurochemical disease. *Int J Obes Relat Metab Disord.* Jan 2004; 28(1):34–38.

Bray GA, Champagne CM. Beyond energy balance: there is more to obesity than kilocalories. *J Am Diet Assoc.* May 2005;105(5 Suppl 1):S17–S23.

CDC. Centers for Disease Control and Prevention. Overweight and obesity: economic consequences. 2011; http://www.cdc.gov/nccdphp/dnpa/obesity/economic_consequences.htm. Accessed July 20, 2011.

Chan JL, Bullen J, Lee JH, Yiannakouris N, Mantzoros CS. Ghrelin levels are not regulated by recombinant leptin administration and/or three days of fasting in healthy subjects. *J Clin Endocrinol Metab.* Jan 2004;89(1):335–343.

Cohen-Cole E, Fletcher JM. Is obesity contagious? Social networks vs. environmental factors in the obesity epidemic. *J Health Econ.* Sep 2008;27(5): 1382–1387.

Cummings DE, Purnell JQ, Frayo RS, Schmidova K, Wisse BE, Weigle DS. A preprandial rise in plasma ghrelin levels suggests a role in meal initiation in humans. *Diabetes.* Aug 2001;50(8):1714–1719.

Cummings DE, Schwartz MW. Genetics and pathophysiology of human obesity. *Annu Rev Med.* 2003;54: 453–471.

Daniels SR, Arnett DK, Eckel RH, et al. Overweight in children and adolescents: pathophysiology, consequences, prevention, and treatment. *Circulation.* Apr 19 2005;111(15):1999–2012.

DiMeglio DP, Mattes RD. Liquid versus solid carbohydrate: effects on food intake and body weight. *Int J Obes Relat Metab Disord.* Jun 2000;24(6):794–800.

Drewnowski A. Obesity, diets, and social inequalities. *Nutr Rev.* May 2009;67 Suppl 1:S36–S39.

ERS. Agriculture Research Service. Food Availability (Per Capita) Data System. 2012; http://www.ers.usda.gov/. Accessed June 30, 2011.

Farley TA, Baker ET, Futrell L, Rice JC. The ubiquity of energy-dense snack foods: a national multicity study. *Am J Public Health.* Feb 2010;100(2):306–311.

Frankenfield DC, Rowe WA, Smith JS, Cooney RN. Validation of several established equations for resting metabolic rate in obese and nonobese people. *J Am Diet Assoc.* Sep 2003;103(9):1152–1159.

Friedman JM. Leptin, leptin receptors, and the control of body weight. *Nutr Rev.* Feb 1998;56(2 Pt 2):s38–s46; discussion s54–s75.

Friedman JM. Obesity: causes and control of excess body fat. *Nature.* May 21 2009;459(7245):340–342.

Glandt M, Raz I. Present and future: pharmacologic treatment of obesity. *J Obes.* 2011. http://www.ncbi.nlm.nih.gov/entrez/query.fcgi?cmd=Retrieve&db=PubMed&dopt=Citation&list_uids=21331293.

Guthrie JF, Morton JF. Food sources of added sweeteners in the diets of Americans. *J Am Diet Assoc.* Jan 2000; 100(1):43–51, quiz 49–50.

Halton TL, Hu FB. The effects of high protein diets on thermogenesis, satiety and weight loss: a critical review. *J Am Coll Nutr.* Oct 2004;23(5):373–385.

Hansen TK, Dall R, Hosoda H, et al. Weight loss increases circulating levels of ghrelin in human obesity. *Clin Endocrinol (Oxf).* Feb 2002;56(2):203–206.

Henry CJ, Emery B. Effect of spiced food on metabolic rate. *Hum Nutr Clin Nutr.* Mar 1986;40(2):165–168.

Heymsfield SB, Greenberg AS, Fujioka K, et al. Recombinant leptin for weight loss in obese and lean adults: a randomized, controlled, dose-escalation trial. *JAMA.* Oct 27 1999;282(16):1568–1575.

Hu FB, Leitzmann MF, Stampfer MJ, Colditz GA, Willett WC, Rimm EB. Physical activity and television watching in relation to risk for type 2 diabetes mellitus in men. *Arch Intern Med.* Jun 25 2001;161(12): 1542–1548.

Johnson L, Mander AP, Jones LR, Emmett PM, Jebb SA. Is sugar-sweetened beverage consumption associated with increased fatness in children? *Nutrition.* Jul–Aug 2007;23(7–8):557–563.

Lantz PM, House JS, Lepkowski JM, Williams DR, Mero RP, Chen J. Socioeconomic factors, health behaviors, and mortality: results from a nationally representative prospective study of US adults. *JAMA.* Jun 3 1998;279(21):1703–1708.

Lowell BB, Spiegelman BM. Towards a molecular understanding of adaptive thermogenesis. *Nature.* Apr 6 2000;404(6778):652–660.

McArdle W, Katch, FL, Katch, VL, eds. *Exercise Physiology: Energy, Nutrition, and Human Performance.* 4th ed. Baltimore, MD: Williams & Wilkins; 1996.

McCrory MA, Fuss PJ, Hays NP, Vinken AG, Greenberg AS, Roberts SB. Overeating in America: association between restaurant food consumption and body fatness in healthy adult men and women ages 19 to 80. *Obes Res.* Nov 1999;7(6):564–571.

Mifflin MD, St Jeor ST, Hill LA, Scott BJ, Daugherty SA, Koh YO. A new predictive equation for resting energy expenditure in healthy individuals. *Am J Clin Nutr.* Feb 1990;51(2):241–247.

Morton GJ, Cummings DE, Baskin DG, Barsh GS, Schwartz MW. Central nervous system control of food intake and body weight. *Nature.* Sep 21 2006;443(7109): 289–295.

Nguyen VT, Larson DE, Johnson RK, Goran MI. Fat intake and adiposity in children of lean and obese parents. *Am J Clin Nutr.* Apr 1996;63(4):507–513.

Ravussin E, Bogardus C. Energy expenditure in the obese: is there a thrifty gene? *Infusionstherapie.* Apr 1990; 17(2):108–112.

Ravussin E, Bogardus C. A brief overview of human energy metabolism and its relationship to essential obesity. *Am J Clin Nutr.* Jan 1992;55(1 Suppl): 242S–245S.

Robinson SM, Jaccard C, Persaud C, Jackson AA, Jequier E, Schutz Y. Protein turnover and thermogenesis in response to high-protein and high-carbohydrate feeding in men. *Am J Clin Nutr.* Jul 1990;52(1):72–80.

Rothwell NJ, Stock MJ. Regulation of energy balance. *Annu Rev Nutr.* 1981;1:235–256.

Schulz LO, Bennett PH, Ravussin E, et al. Effects of traditional and western environments on prevalence of type 2 diabetes in Pima Indians in Mexico and the U.S. *Diabetes Care.* Aug 2006;29(8):1866–1871.

Seagle HM, Strain GW, Makris A, Reeves RS. Position of the American Dietetic Association: weight management. *J Am Diet Assoc.* Feb 2009;109(2):330–346.

Stunkard AJ, Sorensen TI, Hanis C, et al. An adoption study of human obesity. *N Engl J Med.* Jan 23 1986;314(4): 193–198.

USDA-ERS. Food CPI, Prices and Expenditures: Food Expenditures by Families and Individuals as a Share of Disposable Personal Income. 2007; http://www.ers.usda.gov/briefing/cpifoodandexpenditures/Data/Expenditures_tables/table7.htm. Accessed June 10, 2011

Variyam JN. The Price is Right: Economics and the Rise in Obesity. AmberWaves 2005(February, 2005). http://www.ers.usda.gov/AmberWaves/February05/Features/ThePriceIsRight.htm.

Vartanian LR, Schwartz MB, Brownell KD. Effects of soft drink consumption on nutrition and health: a systematic review and meta-analysis. *Am J Public Health.* Apr 2007;97(4):667–675.

Wajchenberg BL. Subcutaneous and visceral adipose tissue: their relation to the metabolic syndrome. *Endocr Rev.* Dec 2000;21(6):697–738.

Westerterp KR. Diet induced thermogenesis. *Nutr Metab (Lond).* Aug 18 2004;1(1):5.

Woods SC. Gastrointestinal satiety signals I. An overview of gastrointestinal signals that influence food intake. *Am J Physiol Gastrointest Liver Physiol.* Jan 2004; 286(1):G7–G13.

Zheng H, Berthoud HR. Neural systems controlling the drive to eat: mind versus metabolism. *Physiology (Bethesda).* Apr 2008;23:75–83.

CHAPTER 4

HEALTH AND ECONOMIC CONSEQUENCES OF OBESITY

READER OBJECTIVES

- Describe medical, psychosocial, and economic consequences associated with obesity
- Explain the metabolic bases and consequences of obesity with an emphasis on the major comorbidities
- Recognize health benefits associated with weight reduction
- Explain the controversies about obesity and reduced longevity
- Understand the role of antiobesity bias and discrimination among the general public and health professionals
- Discuss individual and community economic consequences of obesity

CHAPTER OUTLINE

Health and Economic Consequences of Obesity

The primary concern of overweight and obesity is one of health and not appearance.

—Declaration from the Office of the Surgeon General of the United States (USDHHS, 2007)

The many health consequences of obesity as shown in **Table 4.1** range from biomechanical alterations that cause disability to chronic metabolic abnormalities to an increased risk of premature death. Overweight and obesity increases the risk for dozens of major diseases such as type 2 diabetes, heart disease, hypertension, respiratory problems, osteoarthritis, gallbladder disease, as well as certain types of cancer (NHLBI, 1998). Obesity also has serious psychosocial consequences, such as poor health-related quality of life, low self-esteem, and clinical depression (Sturm, 2001).

TABLE 4.1 Health Consequences of Obesity

Coronary heart disease

Type 2 diabetes

Cancers, such as endometrial, breast, and colon

High blood pressure (hypertension)

High total cholesterol or high levels of triglycerides (dyslipidemia)

Stroke

Liver and gallbladder disease

Sleep apnea and respiratory problems

Degeneration of cartilage and underlying bone within a joint (osteoarthritis)

Reproductive health complications

Modified from: Obesity, Halting the Epidemic by Making Health Easier: At A Glance 2010.
http://www.cdc.gov/chronicdisease/resources/publications/aag/obesity.htm.

Characteristics of Obesity Comorbidities

According to a report on the effect of obesity on health outcomes (Dixon, 2010), three features are necessary to classify a disease as a **comorbidity**, or coexisting condition, of obesity:

1. An Increase in Frequency and Severity of the Disease Occurs When Adiposity Is Present

Clinical and epidemiological studies have shown that, in general, the more obese the individual, the greater the risk for chronic medical conditions associated with excess fat stores. The incidence of heart disease (heart attack, congestive heart failure, sudden cardiac death, and angina or chest pain) is increased with obesity (USDHHS, 2007). A study of more than 2,000 obese adults found that only 9% of women and 12.8% of men had no obesity-related comorbidities (Kannel, 2002). Obesity has been described by the World Health Organization as a condition, prevalent in both developed and developing countries, which is replacing the more traditional public health concerns, such as undernutrition and infectious diseases, as a key contributor to poor health (WHO, 2011).

2. An Improvement or Resolution of the Disease Occurs with Weight Loss

Studies have shown that as little as 5 to 15% loss of total body weight in a person who is overweight or obese reduces the risk factors for conditions such as hypertension and type 2 diabetes (NHLBI, 1998).

3. A Plausible Explanation Exists for the Association of Obesity with the Disease State

Obesity is a condition of chronic energy overload that causes dysfunction through biomechanical alterations associated with increased body weight on organs and joints and also through the interaction of hormones and **cytokines** (signaling molecules) produced by fat cells (Schelbert, 2009). Obesity-related cytokine production generates a state of low-level **chronic systemic inflammation**

FIGURE **4.1**   **Medical complications of obesity.**

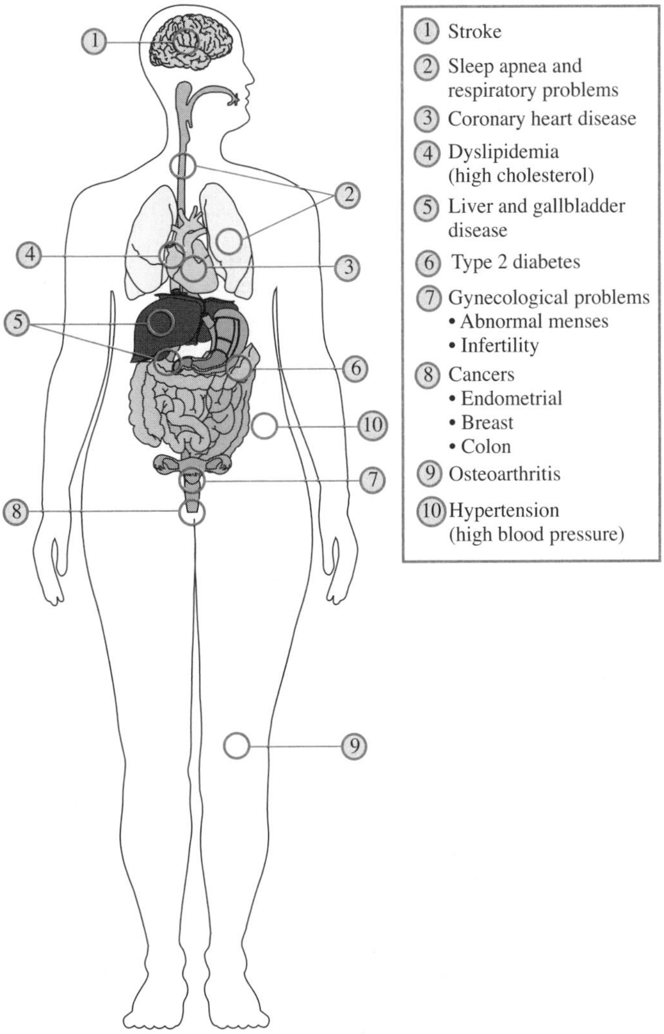

① Stroke
② Sleep apnea and
   respiratory problems
③ Coronary heart disease
④ Dyslipidemia
   (high cholesterol)
⑤ Liver and gallbladder
   disease
⑥ Type 2 diabetes
⑦ Gynecological problems
   • Abnormal menses
   • Infertility
⑧ Cancers
   • Endometrial
   • Breast
   • Colon
⑨ Osteoarthritis
⑩ Hypertension
   (high blood pressure)

Modified from: CDC Obesity and Overweight - Causes and Consequences. http://www.cdc.gov/obesity/adult/causes/index.html.
Organs: © siart/ShutterStock, Inc. Outline: © Anna Rassadnikova/ShutterStock, Inc.

(Tilg, 2006). **Figure 4.1** shows how diverse body systems are affected by obesity.

Following is a discussion of common comorbidities associated with obesity. Sources for more information about these and other conditions linked with obesity are listed in the Resources section.

Obesity and Metabolic Syndrome

The relationship of obesity to metabolic dysfunction does not lie solely in BMI measurement, but rather in the degree of abdominal adiposity. Based on studies using magnetic resonance imaging, it is visceral fat in particular that is correlated with the inflammatory and metabolic disturbances that lead to endocrine, cardiovascular, and malignant consequences (Despres, 2008). Abdominal fat deposition has been associated with **insulin resistance**, a reduced sensitivity to the action of the hormone insulin in processes such as cell glucose uptake, fat metabolism, and control of glucose production by the liver. Insulin resistance results in elevated levels of insulin in the blood, and the hormone may be the link that ties central fat to increased disease risk. Insulin resistance syndrome, commonly called cardiometabolic syndrome or **metabolic syndrome (MetS)**, is a constellation of conditions that increases the risk for type 2 diabetes, heart disease, and **stroke**. **Table 4.2** illustrates how an individual diagnosed with MetS has three or more of these five risk factors: abdominal obesity, elevated blood pressure, low HDL cholesterol, elevated blood triglycerides, and abnormal blood glucose homeostasis.

A person with MetS has approximately twice the risk for coronary heart disease and five times the risk for type 2 diabetes (Grundy, 2005). It is estimated about one-third of adults in the United States now have MetS. That segment of the population includes nearly 55% of adults older than 60 years and 65% of obese Americans. Mexican Americans have the highest prevalence of metabolic syndrome, followed by whites and blacks (Ford, 2002; Ervin, 2009).

Nonalcoholic Fatty Liver Disease

Obesity and insulin resistance increase the risk of nonalcoholic fatty liver disease (NAFLD). This is a condition that encompasses a wide spectrum of liver pathology ranging from **steatosis** (excess fat storage in the liver) to liver inflammation (also called nonalcoholic **steatohepatitis** or NASH), to **cirrhosis**, and liver cancer. About one-third of the US population may have NAFLD, and the disorder is the leading cause of chronic liver disease in the United States (Abdelmalek, 2007). NAFLD resembles alcoholic liver disease but occurs in people who do not overconsume alcohol and most often strikes people who are overweight or obese with elevated blood lipids and diabetes or abnormal blood glucose levels. However, NAFLD can occur without any apparent risk factor in individuals

TABLE 4.2	American Heart Association Adult Treatment Panel III Definition of Metabolic Syndrome
Factor	**Three or more of the following**
Abdominal obesity	Waist circumference: > 40 in. (or 102 cm) for men > 35 in. (or 88 cm) for women
Triglycerides, mg/dl	> 150 mg/dl or on drug treatment for high TG
HDL, mg/dl	< 40 mg/dl for men and < 50 mg/dl for women, or on drug treatment for low HDL
Blood pressure, mmHg	Systolic blood pressure (SBP) > 130 mmHg or diastolic blood pressure > 85 mmHg, or on drug treatment for HTN
Fasting glucose, mg/dl	FPG > 100 mg/dl

FPG: fasting plasma glucose; HDL: high-density lipoprotein; HTN: hypertension; TG: triglycerides.

Data from: Grundy SM. Metabolic syndrome scientific statement by the American Heart Association and the National Heart, Lung, and Blood Institute. *Arterioscler Thromb Vasc Biol.* Nov 2005;25(11):2243–2244.

who are not obese, do not have diabetes, and have normal cholesterol and triglycerides. While the underlying cause of NAFLD is not clear, several factors are possible contributors to the condition (NIDDC, 2006):

- Insulin resistance.
- Release of toxic inflammatory signals by fat cells.
- Oxidative stress that causes damage to liver cells.

While the most common treatment goal for NAFLD is to increase insulin sensitivity with medication or various weight reduction measures including diet, exercise, drug, or surgical therapy, there is currently no scientifically proven therapy to prevent the disease or to avoid its progression.

Polycystic Ovary Syndrome

Polycystic ovary syndrome (PCOS) is a group of metabolic abnormalities associated with insulin resistance, type 2 diabetes, and obesity. PCOS is the most common hormonal disorder among women of reproductive age. It affects up to 10% of women and is associated with infertility, acne, **hirsutism** and increased cardiovascular and cancer risk. The name of the condition comes from the appearance of the ovaries in many women with the disorder. They are enlarged and contain numerous small cysts (Glueck, 2003).

Type 2 Diabetes

Along with the rise in prevalence of obesity and the metabolic syndrome a dramatic increase in type 2 diabetes mellitus has occurred. Diabetes mellitus, or simply diabetes, is a group of diseases characterized by high blood glucose levels (hyperglycemia) that result from defects in production and/or use of insulin. Insulin is a hormone produced by the beta cells of the pancreas that controls the amount of glucose in the blood. In type 2 diabetes, once known as adult-onset or noninsulin-dependent diabetes, either the body does not produce enough insulin or cells are resistant to the effects of insulin. The resulting chronic abnormal blood glucose levels, or hyperglycemia, can give rise to complications that can be life threatening. It is a progressive disease that affects multiple organs and is the most common cause for adult blindness, limb amputations, and kidney failure as well as the leading independent risk factor for coronary artery disease (NIDDK, 2008).

Type 2 diabetes is a comorbidity that is closely linked to obesity. Over 80% of people with the condition are overweight or obese. With a weight gain of 11 to 18 lb a person's risk of developing type 2 diabetes increases to twice that of individuals who have not gained weight (USDHHS, 2007). An investigation of female registered nurses revealed that, while a weight gain of 5 to 7 kg (11 to 15 lb) increased the risk of type 2 diabetes by 50%, losing as little as 5 kg (11 lb) reduced the risk by the same amount (Colditz, 1995).

In the United States the incidence of type 2 diabetes has doubled over the past three decades, most dramatically during the 1990s, among individuals with a BMI of 30 or more. Although the disease may affect people of any age, size, or ethnicity, the disease occurs most often in older people, in African-Americans, American Indians, Native Hawaiians, and other Pacific Islander Americans, Hispanics/Latinos, and non-Hispanic blacks who are overweight and inactive (NIDDK, 1995). Given these statistics, health researchers suggest that type 2 diabetes prevalence in the United States is likely to increase for several reasons:

- Americans are increasingly overweight and sedentary.
- A large segment of the population is aging.
- Hispanics/Latinos and other minority groups at increased risk make up the fastest-growing segment of the United States population.

Another serious concern is that type 2 diabetes has been primarily a disease of adulthood that now occurs with increasing frequency in adolescents. Similar to adults, adolescents with type 2 diabetes have an increased risk for cardiovascular disease. Therefore, adverse events, such as heart attack or stroke, may occur earlier in the life span, perhaps in the third or fourth decade of life (Daniels, 2005).

According to estimates from government agencies, type 2 diabetes will affect one in three people born in 2000 in the United States, and the prevalence of diagnosed diabetes in the United States will increase as much as 165% by 2050 (NIDDK, 2008). The increasing incidence of type 2 diabetes globally is also of serious concern. The disease affects more than 170 million people worldwide. In 2000 the occurrence of type 2 diabetes was greatest in India (40 million), followed by China (21 million), and the United States (18 million). Experts with the World Health Organization have projected that deaths associated with the condition are likely to increase by more than 50% in the next 10 years if the current trajectory continues (WHO, 2011).

BOX 4.1 Healthy Obesity?

All obese individuals do not display increased metabolic and cardiovascular risk factors, just as not all lean individuals are metabolically healthy and disease free. Metabolically healthy but obese (MHO) persons do not show traditional risk factors associated with the insulin resistance syndrome despite having a high accumulation of body fat. As much as 20% of the obese population may be in this category (Karelis, 2004). The higher levels of insulin sensitivity in MHO individuals may be due in part to less distribution of excess fat to the abdominal area. Compared with obese postmenopausal women with the metabolic syndrome, MHO individuals showed 49% less visceral adipose tissue (as measured with **computed tomography**) despite similar levels of total body fatness (Brochu, 2001). This finding supports other studies that suggest that the amount of visceral fat is an important factor associated with insulin resistance (Despres, 2008).

Other studies have shown that middle-aged obese men and women who did not have hypertension, dyslipidemia, or type 2 diabetes were not at increased risk of morbidity or mortality from cardiovascular disease over 10 to 11 years of follow-up compared with normal weight or non-obese individuals (Katzmarzyk, 2006; Song, 2007). Based on this research it might be possible that moderate reduction of visceral body fat through calorie-restricted diets, increased physical activity, or bariatric surgery could transform unhealthy metabolic processes to a healthier state, even if obesity still existed.

Cardiovascular Disease

Cardiovascular disease (CVD) is the leading chronic disease in the United States. CVD generally refers to conditions that involve narrowed or blocked blood vessels that can initiate a heart attack, chest pain, or stroke. The risk for CVD is increased by a number of factors, including hypertension, abnormal blood lipids such as low **high-density lipoproteins (HDL)**, elevated **low-density lipoproteins (LDL)**, and inflammation. As obesity is associated with these disorders, it is a primary contributor to heart disease. As shown in **Figure 4.2**, as BMI increases the prevalence of low HDL-cholesterol levels increases in both women and men. Low HDL was defined here as < 35 mg/dL in men and < 45 mg/dL in women.

Of the influences of obesity on CVD, the disorder with the closest association is hypertension, a condition that is twice as common in adults who are obese as for those who are at a healthy weight (USDHHS, 2007). In **Figure 4.3**,

data from NHANES III show that the prevalence of hypertension (mean systolic pressure ≥ 140 and/ or diastolic pressure ≥ 90 mm Hg) increases progressively with higher levels of BMI in men and women. The prevalence in adults with BMI > 30 is 41.9% for men and 37.8% for women compared with 14.9% for men and 15.2% for women with BMI ≤ 25.

Obesity also presents an unexplained paradox in relation to CVD. Studies have reported that obese patients with CVD have improved survival rates compared with patients with ideal body weight. Individuals in the overweight (BMI 25–29.9) category had the lowest risk for CVD, and obese stage I patients (BMI 30–35) had no increased risk for total mortality. Obesity alone is not a major predictor of death from CVD once other risk factors that correlate with obesity have been removed (Romero-Corral, 2006). For example, an obese person with normal values for blood pressure and serum lipids is not at increased risk. The most important issue is not extra weight in itself but rather

FIGURE 4.2 Prevalence of low HDL-cholesterol according to BMI by sex.

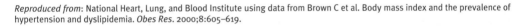

Reproduced from: National Heart, Lung, and Blood Institute using data from Brown C et al. Body mass index and the prevalence of hypertension and dyslipidemia. *Obes Res*. 2000;8:605–619.

FIGURE 4.3 Prevalence of hypertension according to BMI.

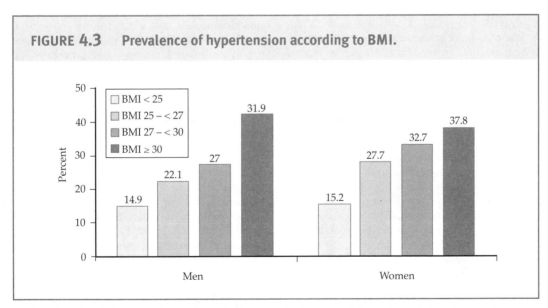

Reproduced from: National Heart, Lung, and Blood Institute using data from Brown C et al. Body mass index and the prevalence of hypertension and dyslipidemia. *Obes Res*. 2000;8:605–619.

the metabolic consequences that may occur along with obesity (Poirer, 2006).

Respiratory Disease

Obesity is a strong predictor of respiratory disorders such as **obstructive sleep apnea** and **asthma**. Breathing problems associated with obesity are thought to occur due to mechanical issues or increased inflammatory response.

Obstructive Sleep Apnea

Obstructive sleep apnea (OSA) is caused by a blockage of the airway, usually when the soft tissue in the rear of the throat collapses and closes during sleep. This condition causes repeated interrupted breathing, sometimes hundreds of times, during a sleep period. Symptoms of OSA consist of excessive daytime sleepiness, problems with memory and concentration, and increased risk of hypertension. OSA may be responsible for poor performance at work, motor vehicle accidents, and academic underachievement in children and adolescents (NHLBI, 2010). Upper-body obesity and a large neck circumference in both men and women are highly predictive of OSA. Men with a neck circumference of 17 in. or greater and women whose neck circumference is 16 in. or more are at high risk for OSA (Davies, 1990). Most people with OSA have a BMI > 30 and moderate weight loss can significantly improve the symptoms (Malnick, 2006).

Asthma

Asthma is a disease characterized by recurrent attacks of breathlessness and wheezing, which vary in severity from mild to life threatening. In an asthma attack, the lining of the passages swell, causing the airways to narrow and reduce the flow of air in and out of the lungs. Potential mechanisms for this relationship between asthma and obesity include restriction in lung volume and adipocyte-related systemic inflammation that could contribute to airway hyperresponsiveness that adversely affects airway smooth muscle function causing constriction and airway narrowing (Malnick, 2006). Epidemiologic studies have shown an increased prevalence of asthma in people with obesity and the association that is especially strong among women. When obese asthma patients re-

duce weight asthma symptoms are often improved (Ford, 2005).

Malignancies

A population study in the United States of more than 900,000 adults estimated that 14% of deaths from cancer in men and 20% of deaths in women were due to overweight and obesity (Calle, 2003). Obesity is associated with an increased risk for some types of cancer, particularly the hormone-dependent and gastrointestinal cancers. Those include endometrial (cancer of the lining of the uterus), colon, prostate, and breast cancer. Women who gain more than 20 lb after age 18 double their risk of postmenopausal breast cancer, compared to women whose weight remains stable (NHLBI, 1998). The biologic mechanism that explains how obesity increases cancer risk may be different for different cancers. Possible explanations associated with increased body fat implicate alterations in sex hormones and increased levels of oxidative stress, which may be linked to DNA mutation and abnormal cell growth as is seen in many types of cancer. At this time, there is no good evidence that intentional weight loss affects risk for any cancer (Trentham-Dietz, 2000). This reality lends further support to the benefit of weight gain prevention for general health as well as the possibly that initiation of certain types of cancers will be reduced.

Musculoskeletal Disorders

There is a positive association between musculoskeletal disorders, physical disability, and level of obesity. Obesity may have a substantial effect on musculoskeletal pain and injury in the back, hip, knee, ankle, and foot because of the stress placed on the tendons, cartilage, and joints by extra weight. In addition, biomechanical adaptations in response to increased fat mass and altered center of gravity affect locomotion, balance, and strength (Wearing, 2006). A strong relationship also exists between obesity and the development and progression of osteoarthritis, especially in women. **Osteoarthritis (OA)** is the most common joint disorder and is a primary cause of disability among adults. The disease is characterized by a degeneration of cartilage and underlying bone within a joint that eventually leads to pain and stiffness. The areas most commonly affected are the knees, hips, and joints in the hands and spine. For every 2-lb increase in weight, the risk of developing OA is increased by 9 to 13%. Symptoms often improve with weight loss (USDHHS, 2007). The specific causes of OA are unknown, but a combination of both mechanical and metabolic factors may be responsible. The fact that OA frequently occurs in non-weight-bearing joints suggests there are components of obesity or excess adipose tissue that alter cartilage and bone metabolism independent of increased body weight (Malnick, 2006).

Longevity

In 2003 Surgeon General Richard Carmona announced to the United States House of Representatives, "I welcome this chance to talk with you about a health crisis affecting every State, every city, every community, and every school across our great Nation. The crisis is obesity. It's the fastest growing cause of death in America" (Carmona, 2003). Although life expectancy has been increasing in the United States population (NCHS, 2009), some investigators suggest that, in the near future, the trend may reverse because of the numerous comorbid disorders associated with excess body fat. As a result of the increase in childhood obesity, conditions that were once considered adult diseases such as type 2 diabetes, hypertension, CVD, and joint deterioration are more often being diagnosed in children. For the first time in history, the next generation may not live longer than their parents (Olshansky, 2005).

As would be expected for a condition that increases the risk of serious medical conditions, obesity increases the risk of premature mortality. It has been estimated that as many as 300,000 deaths per year in the United States are due to obesity (Flegal, 2005). A study of more than 40,000 overweight women with obesity-related conditions found that any amount of weight loss was associated with a 20% reduction in all-cause death (Williamson, 1995). The relationship between BMI and mortality, which varies with ethnicity and age, is generally a J-shaped curve with increased mortality at both lower and higher numbers. In an analysis of data from almost 900,000 adults, mostly in Western Europe and North America, overall mortality was

lowest at a BMI ≥ 22.5 to 25 in both sexes and at all ages (Whitlock, 2009). In another analysis overweight (BMI 25 to ≥ 30) was not associated with excess deaths; however, individuals with a BMI of 30 or greater had a 10 to 50% increased risk of death from all causes, compared with healthy weight individuals (Flegal, 2005). Extreme obesity (BMI ≥ 40) has been estimated to shorten life by 5 to 20 years, depending on sex, age, and ethnic group (Fontaine, 2003). The relative increased risk of obesity-associated mortality seems to diminish with age, as statistically significant increases in mortality have not been reported in obese adults older than 75 years (Stevens, 1998). At the other end of the spectrum individuals with a very low BMI may be at increased risk. For example, individuals with a BMI less than 18.5 have approximately double the mortality rate of individuals with a BMI between 20 and 25. Because serious health problems such as cancer or infections may cause weight loss, this relationship is not necessarily an indication that low weight in itself causes increased mortality (Flegal, 2007).

Controversies About Obesity and Longevity

While the association of obesity and increased risk of death and disease is generally consistent, the probable number of American lives lost to obesity has been controversial. Estimates of the annual number of deaths attributable to overweight and obesity have ranged from 110,000 to 400,000 depending on the different methods used to correlate mortality and obesity. In the opinion of some scientists, concern over the risks of obesity is overstated. Epidemiological studies reveal that, apart from the extremes, BMI category alone is not a strong predictor of death rates. It may be that more-aggressive treatment of obesity-related diabetes, hypertension, hyperlipidemia, and other metabolic disorders have allowed people to live longer even with these conditions.

Psychosocial Correlates of Obesity

Quality of Life

Because it is such an incapacitating disease, obesity can affect the quality of life (QOL) by limiting mobility and decreasing physical capacity as well as through social, academic, employment, and medical discrimination. A good measure of the success of an obesity treatment might be its effect on an individual's QOL. Overall QOL can be categorized into physical, social, and psychological functional domains.

In the physical domain, obesity is associated with major mobility problems that limit **activities of daily living (ADLs)**. Health professionals assess ability or inability to perform ADLs as a measurement of the functional status of a person, particularly in regard to defining whether or not a person is disabled. Physical constraints can make personal hygiene and cleanliness difficult when simple tasks such as drying oneself after a shower, cutting toenails, or tying shoelaces become major logistical tasks. Obese women reported that their main mobility aggravations were associated with strain and pain at work, walking outdoors, managing stairs, and getting up from low chairs. They also reported difficulty with housework that requires squatting, stooping, or lifting (Larsson, 2001).

Discrimination and Bias

The social domain of QOL is affected by weight discrimination and bias that is rarely challenged, and stereotyping of obese persons is common in the United States. Negative attitudes and bias toward obese persons have been frequently reported by employers, coworkers, teachers, peers, friends, family members, and healthcare workers, perhaps because weight stigma remains a socially acceptable from of bias (Cramer, 1998; Puhl, 2007). Jokes and derogatory portrayals are common in the popular media. Numerous studies have documented harmful weight-based stereotypes that overweight and obese individuals are lazy, weak-willed, unsuccessful, unintelligent, lack self-discipline, have poor willpower, and are noncompliant with weight-loss treatment (Puhl, 2009). Surveys indicate that coworkers and employers view obese employees as less competent and lacking in self-discipline. These attitudes can have a negative impact on wages, promotions, and hiring for obese employees. Other studies show that obese applicants are less likely to be hired than thinner applicants, despite having identical job qualifications (Puhl, 2009). With the prevailing

societal attitudes, obese individuals are blamed for their excess weight, and weight stigmatization is justified because obese individuals are perceived as being personally responsible for their weight. Stigma and ridicule may even be seen as a useful way to motivate obese persons to adopt healthier lifestyles (Puhl, 2003).

Many forms of weight stigmatization occur in school settings. Obese students face numerous obstacles, including harassment and rejection from peers. Research shows that stigma toward overweight students begins early. Negative attitudes have been reported among preschool children (ages 3 to 5) who said overweight peers were mean, stupid, ugly, unhappy, lazy, and had few friends (Puhl, 2001). A primary factor that mediates adverse psychosocial effects of obesity is compromised peer relationships (Strauss, 2003). Various reports indicate that overweight children have fewer friends and those friendships are often isolated or peripheral relationships. In addition to having fewer friends, being teased about weight is another important indicator of psychosocial distress. Obese children are more likely to be bullied regardless of sex, race, socioeconomic status (SES), or academic achievement (Lumeng, 2010). It has been shown that obese youth who have been subjected to teasing report an increase in both thoughts of suicide and number of suicide attempts (Eisenberg, 2003). Adolescents who are overweight are less likely to marry, complete fewer years of education, and have a lower household income in adulthood (Haas, 2003).

Weight stigma also exists in healthcare settings. Obese patients may be reluctant to seek medical care, and are more likely to delay preventive healthcare services and cancel medical appointments. These incidents may happen as a way to avoid facing weight bias from healthcare providers (Phul, 2010). Physicians, nurses, dietitians, psychologists, and medical students have reported negative attitudes about overweight patients. In one study, health professionals and researchers attending an international obesity conference had similar antiobesity biases as the general public. They endorsed the stereotypes of fat people being lazy, stupid, and worthless. Their attitudes and behaviors reflect a view held by people who are not healthcare professionals: If individuals would simply eat less and exercise more, they would not be obese (Schwartz, 2003). There is other evidence that healthcare professionals who specialize in the treatment of obesity hold negative attitudes as well. Reports show that many associate obesity and overweight with poor hygiene, dishonesty, family problems, a lack of intelligence, inactivity, and a lack of will power. Furthermore, some of these professionals spent less time with overweight patients and indicated they preferred not to treat or touch these patients and were repulsed by them (Ruelaz, 2007).

Psychological Implications

The consequences of being denied jobs, rejected by peers, or treated inappropriately by healthcare professionals because of one's weight can lead to a number of psychological problems. Obese women have reported that they avoided certain situations such as air travel because of anxiety over seating difficulties, and they felt embarrassed to take part in their children's activities (Wadden, 2006; Dixon, 2010). Other obesity-related mental health disorders include depression and low self-esteem (Kottke, 2003). In particular, people with extreme obesity have been found to be more likely to have a lower sense of self-worth and fewer close relationships than people in the less extreme classes of obesity. In a study exploring the relationship between obesity and depression, morbidly obese women were nearly four times more likely to have experienced major depression in the month preceding the study than women of normal weight (Onyike, 2003). Those who were obese as children are more likely to be unhappy with their physical appearance and to have lower self-esteem than those who became obese as adults (Wardle, 2002). As with other obesity-related comorbidities, there is generally a marked improvement in psychological symptoms with substantial weight loss (Dixon, 2010). Providing another point of view, there are also numerous studies in which authors caution against assuming that all obese women are depressed or have mood disorders. Being exposed to bias and discrimination doesn't necessarily translate into psychological problems (Jackson, 2000).

Given how pervasive weight stigma is in our society, transforming attitudes and enforcing laws that prohibit discrimination based on weight are necessary to decrease the problem of bias. There are a number of organizations that are trying to end discrimination against obese people. One example is the National Association to Advance Fat Acceptance (NAAFA), which was founded in1997. The NAAFA goal is to help build a society in which people of every size are accepted with dignity and equality in all aspects of life. Another group, Health at Every Size (HAES), supports a movement based on the belief that healthy bodies come in all sizes and shapes. Their philosophy extends the simple premise that the best way to improve health is to honor the body. It encourages adopting health habits for the sake of health and well-being rather than weight control. Sources for more information about these organizations can be found in the Resources section in this chapter.

Economic Costs of Obesity

Health issues associated with overweight and obesity have a significant economic impact on individuals and the United States healthcare system. Researchers at the CDC estimated that the costs of treating obese individuals in 2008, paid by Medicare, Medicaid, and private insurers, was $147 billion and accounted for nearly 10% of all medical spending in the United States (Finkelstein, 2009). The economic burden on society of obesity-related illness is measured in terms of direct and indirect costs. Direct costs refer to preventive, diagnostic, and treatment services such as physician visits, medications, and hospital and nursing home care. High direct costs come from increased frequency of doctor visits, more expensive treatments, more hospitalization as well as higher drug costs that are associated with obesity. These costs are not due to obesity alone, but to the cancer, heart disease, type 2 diabetes, arthritis, and other diseases that are associated with obesity. These expenditures represent the value of resources that could be allocated to other uses in the absence of disease (NHLBI, 1998). Indirect costs occur when people are unable to work and do not receive wages because of illness or disability. These costs account for the value of reduction or cessation of productivity and lost future earnings.

The increase in numbers of patients in the extremely obese category also puts a different type of strain on the healthcare system. Lifting injuries among physical therapists, nurses, and other healthcare workers are increasing (Tizer, 2007). There are new hospital expenditures for special beds, scales, operating tables, stretchers, remodeling structures for wider doorways, installing overhead hoists, and converting wall-mounted toilets to floor-mounted ones. In many medical practices there is a need for larger gowns and linens and wheelchairs that will stand up to the weight of very heavy patients. In addition to healthcare costs, expenditures related to the pharmaceutical, fitness, diet, and fashion industries are part of the economic impact of obesity.

The costs associated with various obesity treatments must be balanced with potential outcomes. A weight loss of as little as 5 to 10% may produce substantial health benefits such as lowering blood pressure, blood glucose, and triglycerides. Such health improvements could offset the costs of obesity therapy over the long term (NHLBI, 1998). However, without adequate reimbursement, healthcare professionals are hesitant to take on long-term patient obesity management. Some health insurers cover obesity treatment but the coverage is not widespread. The key concern of insurance companies is: Will a large investment in developing and implementing effective obesity treatment and prevention produce an adequate increase in good health and quality of life and a decrease in healthcare costs?

Summary

Obesity is strongly associated with chronic conditions such as type 2 diabetes, cardiovascular diseases including stroke and hypertension, musculoskeletal disorders, some forms of cancer, and even premature death. The rate of adult diseases, such as type 2 diabetes, high blood pressure, and high cholesterol, in children has risen along with the rates of obesity. Studies suggest that the more overweight a person is the more likely they are to have health problems. Among obese individuals the characteristics of adipose tissue, including where it is located and its metabolic activity, may have a greater impact on well-being than the total amount of fat stored. Abdominal obesity is associated with greater risks to health than peripheral fat distribution.

Obesity has an impact on an individual's quality of life (QOL) due to limits on physical mobility and the incidence of bias and discrimination in schools, the workplace, and even in medical treatment. In some people with obesity, psychological implications such as depression, anxiety, and low self-esteem may occur as a result of factors that diminish QOL. Reducing the acceptability and occurrence of bias and discrimination is an important societal goal that could help improve QOL for individuals with obesity.

The cost of obesity and health-related problems may account for as much as 10% of all medical spending in the United States. In addition, there are increased costs of lost productivity and costs for specialized beds, chairs, and equipment required to accommodate larger individuals. Investing in prevention and management of obesity now could be a valuable means of reducing the large economic burden of obesity in the future.

Critical Thinking Questions

Question: What is the significance of visceral fat in the context of these obesity-related diseases?

Metabolic syndrome
Type 2 diabetes
Cardiovascular disease
Respiratory disease
Malignancies

Question: How does visceral fat distribution apply to the concept of a metabolically healthy but obese (MHO) person?

Question: Why is there controversy about the effect of obesity on longevity?

Question: Provide examples of bias and discrimination against individuals with obesity that you have observed in the media and in social or professional settings.

Question: Because there is currently a large percentage of Americans with obesity do you think body size bias and discrimination has been reduced?

Question: Why does obesity cause such a large economic burden? Discuss the impact of both direct and indirect costs.

Resources

American Diabetes Association

http://www.diabetes.org/

Health at Every Size

http://www.haescommunity.org/

Overweight and Obesity: Economic Consequences

http://www.cdc.gov/obesity/causes/economics.html

Overweight and Obesity: Health Consequences

http://www.cdc.gov/obesity/causes/health.html

National Association to Advance Fat Acceptance

http://www.naafaonline.com/dev2/index.html

Vital Signs: Adult Obesity

http://www.cdc.gov/VitalSigns/AdultObesity/index.html

Clinical Guidelines on the Identification, Evaluation, and Treatment of Overweight and Obesity in Adults

http://www.nhlbi.nih.gov/guidelines/obesity/ob_home.htm

This site provides detailed information about health problems associated with overweight and obesity.

References

Abdelmalek MF, Diehl AM. Nonalcoholic fatty liver disease as a complication of insulin resistance. *Med Clin North Am.* Nov 2007;91(6):1125–1149, ix.

Brochu M, Tchernof A, Dionne IJ, et al. What are the physical characteristics associated with a normal metabolic profile despite a high level of obesity in postmenopausal women? *J Clin Endocrinol Metab.* Mar 2001;86(3):1020–1025.

Calle EE, Rodriguez C, Walker-Thurmond K, Thun MJ. Overweight, obesity, and mortality from cancer in a prospectively studied cohort of U.S. adults. *N Engl J Med.* Apr 24 2003;348(w17):1625–1638.

Carmona R. The Obesity Crisis in America Testimony Before the Subcommittee on Education Reform Committee on Education and the Workforce United States House of Representatives. 2003; http://www.surgeongeneral.gov/news/testimony/obesity07162003.htm. Accessed June 20, 2011.

Colditz GA, Willett WC, Rotnitzky A, Manson JE. Weight gain as a risk factor for clinical diabetes mellitus in women. *Ann Intern Med.* Apr 1 1995;122(7): 481–486.

Cramer P, Steinwert, T. Thin is good, fat is bad: how early does it begin? *J Appl Dev Psychol.* 1998;19:429–451.

Daniels SR, Arnett DK, Eckel RH, et al. Overweight in children and adolescents: pathophysiology, consequences, prevention, and treatment. *Circulation.* Apr 19 2005;111(15):1999–2012.

Davies R, Stradling, JR. The relationship between neck circumference, radiographic pharyngeal anatomy, and the obstructive sleep apnoea syndrome. *Eur Respir J.* 1990;3:509–514.

Despres JP, Lemieux I, Bergeron J, et al. Abdominal obesity and the metabolic syndrome: contribution to global cardiometabolic risk. *Arterioscler Thromb Vasc Biol.* Jun 2008;28(6):1039–1049.

Dixon JB. The effect of obesity on health outcomes. *Mol Cell Endocrinol.* Mar 25 2010;316(2):104–108.

Eisenberg ME, Neumark-Sztainer D, Story M. Associations of weight-based teasing and emotional well-being among adolescents. *Arch Pediatr Adolesc Med.* Aug 2003;157(8):733–738.

Ervin RB. Prevalence of metabolic syndrome among adults 20 years of age and over, by sex, age, race and ethnicity, and body mass index: United States, 2003–2006. *Natl Health Stat Report.* May 5 2009;(13):1–7.

Finkelstein EA, Trogdon JG, Cohen JW, Dietz W. Annual medical spending attributable to obesity: payer-and service-specific estimates. *Health Aff (Millwood).* Sep–Oct 2009;28(5):w822–w831.

Flegal KM, Graubard BI, Williamson DF, Gail MH. Excess deaths associated with underweight, overweight, and obesity. *JAMA.* Apr 20 2005;293(15):1861–1867.

Flegal KM, Graubard BI, Williamson DF, Gail MH. Cause-specific excess deaths associated with underweight, overweight, and obesity. *JAMA.* Nov 7 2007;298(17): 2028–2037.

Fontaine KR, Redden DT, Wang C, Westfall AO, Allison DB. Years of life lost due to obesity. *JAMA.* Jan 8 2003; 289(2):187–193.

Ford ES, Giles WH, Dietz WH. Prevalence of the metabolic syndrome among US adults: findings from the third National Health and Nutrition Examination Survey. *JAMA.* Jan 16 2002;287(3):356–359.

Ford ES. The epidemiology of obesity and asthma. *J Allergy Clin Immunol.* May 2005;115(5):897–909; quiz 910.

Glueck CJ, Papanna R, Wang P, Goldenberg N, Sieve-Smith L. Incidence and treatment of metabolic syndrome in newly referred women with confirmed polycystic ovarian syndrome. *Metabolism.* Jul 2003;52(7):908–915.

Grundy SM. Metabolic syndrome scientific statement by the American Heart Association and the National Heart, Lung, and Blood Institute. *Arterioscler Thromb Vasc Biol.* Nov 2005;25(11):2243–2244.

Haas JS, Lee LB, Kaplan CP, Sonneborn D, Phillips KA, Liang SY. The association of race, socioeconomic status, and health insurance status with the prevalence of overweight among children and adolescents. *Am J Public Health.* Dec 2003;93(12):2105–2110.

Jackson TD, Grilo CM, Masheb RM. Teasing history, onset of obesity, current eating disorder psychopathology, body dissatisfaction, and psychological functioning in binge eating disorder. *Obes Res.* Sep 2000;8(6): 451–458.

Kannel WB, Wilson PW, Nam BH, D'Agostino RB. Risk stratification of obesity as a coronary risk factor. *Am J Cardiol.* Oct 1 2002;90(7):697–701.

Karelis AD, St-Pierre DH, Conus F, Rabasa-Lhoret R, Poehlman ET. Metabolic and body composition factors in subgroups of obesity: what do we know? *J Clin Endocrinol Metab.* Jun 2004;89(6): 2569–2575.

Katzmarzyk PT, Janssen I, Ross R, Church TS, Blair SN. The importance of waist circumference in the definition of metabolic syndrome: prospective analyses of mortality in men. *Diabetes Care.* Feb 2006;29(2): 404–409.

Kottke TE, Wu LA, Hoffman RS. Economic and psychological implications of the obesity epidemic. *Mayo Clin Proc.* Jan 2003;78(1):92–94.

Larsson UE, Mattsson E. Perceived disability and observed functional limitations in obese women. *Int J Obes Relat Metab Disord.* Nov 2001;25(11):1705–1712.

Lumeng JC, Forrest P, Appugliese DP, Kaciroti N, Corwyn RF, Bradley RH. Weight status as a predictor of being bullied in third through sixth grades. *Pediatrics.* Jun 2010;125(6):e1301–e1307.

Malnick SD, Knobler H. The medical complications of obesity. *QJM.* Sep 2006;99(9):565–579.

NCHS. Life Expectancy at All Time High; Death Rates Reach New Low, New Report Shows. 2009; http://www.cdc.gov/media/pressrel/2009/r090819.htm. Accessed June 10, 2011.

NHLBI. National Heart, Lung, and Blood Institute. Clinical guidelines on the identification, evaluation, and treatment of overweight and obesity in adults: executive summary. Vol. No. 98–4083. Bethesda, MD: National Institutes of Health; 1998.

NHLBI. National Heart, Lung, and Blood Institute. What Is Sleep Apnea? 2010; http://www.nhlbi.nih.gov/health/dci/Diseases/SleepApnea/SleepApnea_WhatIs.html. Accessed April 10, 2011.

NIDDIC. Nonalcoholic Steatohepatitis. No. 07–4921. 2006; http://digestive.niddk.nih.gov/ddiseases/pubs/nash/. Accessed November 20, 2011.

NIDDK. Diabetes Overview. 2008; http://diabetes.niddk.nih.gov/dm/pubs/overview/. Accessed May 10, 2011.

NIDDK. *Diabetes in America.* No. 95-468. Bethesda, MD: National Institutes of Health; 1995.

Olshansky SJ, Passaro DJ, Hershow RC, et al. A potential decline in life expectancy in the United States in the 21st century. *N Engl J Med.* Mar 17 2005;352(11): 1138–1145.

Onyike CU, Crum RM, Lee HB, Lyketsos CG, Eaton WW. Is obesity associated with major depression? Results from the Third National Health and Nutrition Examination Survey. *Am J Epidemiol.* Dec 15 2003; 158(12):1139–1147.

Poirier P. Recurrent cardiovascular events in contemporary cardiology: obesity patients should not rest in PEACE. *Eur Heart J.* Jun 2006;27(12):1390–1391.

Puhl R, Brownell KD. Bias, discrimination, and obesity. *Obes Res.* Dec 2001;9(12):788–805.

Puhl R, Brownell KD. Ways of coping with obesity stigma: review and conceptual analysis. *Eat Behav.* Mar 2003;4(1):53–78.

Puhl RM, Heuer CA. Obesity stigma: important considerations for public health. *Am J Public Health.* Jun 2010;100(6):1019–1028.

Puhl RM, Heuer CA. The stigma of obesity: a review and update. *Obesity (Silver Spring).* May 2009;17(5): 941–964.

Puhl RM, Latner JD. Stigma, obesity, and the health of the nation's children. *Psychol Bull.* 2007;133(4): 557–580.

Romero-Corral A, Montori VM, Somers VK, et al. Association of bodyweight with total mortality and with cardiovascular events in coronary artery disease: a systematic review of cohort studies. *Lancet.* Aug 19 2006;368(9536):666–678.

Ruelaz AR, Diefenbach P, Simon B, Lanto A, Arterburn D, Shekelle PG. Perceived barriers to weight management in primary care—perspectives of patients and providers. *J Gen Intern Med.* Apr 2007;22(4): 518–522.

Schelbert KB. Comorbidities of obesity. *Prim Care.* Jun 2009; 36(2):271–285.

Schwartz MB, Chambliss HO, Brownell KD, Blair SN, Billington C. Weight bias among health professionals specializing in obesity. *Obes Res.* Sep 2003; 11(9):1033–1039.

Song Y, Manson JE, Meigs JB, Ridker PM, Buring JE, Liu S. Comparison of usefulness of body mass index versus metabolic risk factors in predicting 10-year risk of cardiovascular events in women. *Am J Cardiol.* Dec 1 2007;100(11):1654–1658.

Stevens J, Cai J, Pamuk ER, Williamson DF, Thun MJ, Wood JL. The effect of age on the association between body-mass index and mortality. *N Engl J Med.* Jan 1 1998;338(1):1–7.

Strauss RS, Pollack HA. Social marginalization of overweight children. *Arch Pediatr Adolesc Med.* Aug 2003; 157(8):746–752.

Sturm R, Wells KB. Does obesity contribute as much to morbidity as poverty or smoking? *Public Health.* May 2001;115(3):229–235.

Tilg H, Moschen AR. Adipocytokines: mediators linking adipose tissue, inflammation and immunity. *Nat Rev Immunol.* Oct 2006;6(10):772–783.

Tizer K. Extremely obese patients in the healthcare setting: patient and staff safety. *J Ambul Care Manage.* Apr–Jun 2007;30(2):134–141.

Trentham-Dietz A, Newcomb PA, Egan KM, et al. Weight change and risk of postmenopausal breast cancer (United States). *Cancer Causes Control.* Jul 2000; 11(6):533–542.

USDHHS. U.S. Department of Health and Human Services. *The Surgeon General's call to action to prevent and decrease overweight and obesity.* Rockville, MD: Office of the Surgeon General; 2007.

Wadden TA, Foster GD. Weight and Lifestyle Inventory (WALI). *Obesity (Silver Spring).* Mar 2006;14 Suppl 2: 99S–118S.

Wardle J, Waller J, Fox E. Age of onset and body dissatisfaction in obesity. *Addict Behav.* Jul–Aug 2002;27(4): 561–573.

Wearing SC, Hennig EM, Byrne NM, Steele JR, Hills AP. Musculoskeletal disorders associated with obesity:

a biomechanical perspective. *Obes Rev.* Aug 2006; 7(3):239–250.

Whitlock G, Lewington S, Sherliker P, et al. Body-mass index and cause-specific mortality in 900,000 adults: collaborative analyses of 57 prospective studies. *Lancet.* Mar 28 2009;373(9669):1083–1096.

WHO. World Health Organization. Obesity and Overweight Fact Sheet No. 311. 2011; http://www.who .int/mediacentre/factsheets/fs311/en/. Accessed March 20, 2011.

Williamson DF, Pamuk E, Thun M, Flanders D, Byers T, Heath C. Prospective study of intentional weight loss and mortality in never-smoking overweight US white women aged 40–64 years. *Am J Epidemiol.* Jun 15 1995;141(12):1128–1141.

STRATEGIES AND RESEARCH FOR WEIGHT MANAGEMENT AND OBESITY PREVENTION

CHAPTER 5

DIETARY INTERVENTIONS FOR OBESITY PREVENTION AND MANAGEMENT

READER OBJECTIVES

- Describe and practice methods of determining optimal energy intake for weight management
- Discuss current evidence-based recommendations for choosing healthful food patterns
- Compare the advantages of the 2010 MyPlate plan with the Food Guide Pyramid
- Explain how MyPlate components may facilitate weight management
- Describe how energy density is related to the MyPlate food groups and to solid fats and added sugars
- Summarize results of research studies that compare weight-loss diets
- Interpret the implications of the great variety of diets used by participants in the National Weight Control Registry

CHAPTER OUTLINE

Energy Requirements for Weight Management

Matching the calories consumed from foods and beverages with energy expenditure is essential to achieving and maintaining energy balance. The total number of calories a person needs each day varies depending on age, sex, height, weight, and level of physical activity. In addition, an individual's personal health goal to lose, maintain, or gain weight also affects how many calories should be consumed. **Table 5.1** provides estimated daily calorie needs for weight maintenance.

In general, energy requirements range from 1,600 to 2,400 calories per day for adult women and 2,000 to 3,000 calories per day for adult men. Dietary calorie needs for young children range from 1,000 to 2,000 calories per day. The range for older children and adolescents varies widely from 1,400 to 3,200 calories per day and boys typically have higher calorie needs than girls. These are broad estimates, and individual calorie needs can be more precisely calculated with online tools such as those available on the USDA Dietary Guidelines website. Food labels and numerous books and calorie counting websites (check the Resources section of this chapter) are useful to determine the calories in foods. The easiest and most straightforward way for people to assess whether they are eating the appropriate number of calories is to monitor body weight and adjust calorie intake and physical activity based on how the weight changes over time.

The NHLBI Dietary Guidelines advocate modest weight loss of 10% of body weight with a diet

TABLE 5.1 Calorie Goals at Three Levels of Physical Activity*

Gender	Age (years)	Activity level		
		Sedentary	Moderately active	Active
Child	2–3	1,000	1,000–1,400	1,000–1,400
Female	4–8	1,200	1,400–1,600	1,400–1,800
	9–13	1,600	1,600–2,000	1,800–2,200
	14–18	1,800	2,000	2,400
	19–30	2,000	2,000–2,200	2,400
	31–50	1,800	2,000	2,200
	51+	1,600	1,800	2,000–2,200
Male	4–8	1,400	1,400–1,600	1,600–2,000
	9–13	1,800	1,800–2,200	2,000–2,600
	14–18	2,200	2,400–2,800	2,800–3,200
	19–30	2,400	2,600–2,800	3,000
	31–50	2,200	2,400–2,600	2,800–3,000
	51+	2,000	2,200–2,400	2,400–2,800

Calorie levels are based on Estimated Energy Requirements (EER) from the Institute of Medicine Dietary Reference Intakes macronutrients report, 2002, calculated by gender, age, and activity level for reference-sized individuals.

*Physical activity levels are defined as:

Sedentary includes only the light physical activity associated with typical day-to-day life.

Moderately active includes physical activity equivalent to walking about 1.5 to 3 miles per day at 3 to 4 miles per hour, in addition to the light physical activity associated with typical day-to-day life.

Active includes physical activity equivalent to walking more than 3 miles per day at 3 to 4 miles per hour, in addition to the light physical activity associated with typical day-to-day life.

Source: U.S. Department of Agriculture and U.S. Department of Health and Human Services. Dietary Guidelines for Americans, 2010. 7th Edition, Washington, DC: U.S. Government Printing Office, December 2010, p. 14.

that is based on calorie reduction and is planned to meet an individual's needs and lifestyle (NHLBI, 1998). As a rough estimation, 1 lb of body fat is the result of eating about 3,500 extra calories. Reducing calorie intake by 500 to 1,000 calories per day theoretically results in the loss of 1 to 2 lb of fat per week (Dunn, 2006). For most people this means that a reduced energy plan will total about 1,000 to 1,200 calories for women and 1,200 to 1,600 calories for men. Understanding calorie needs and recognizing food sources of calories are important concepts when creating an eating pattern that supports weight management. Yet most Americans are unaware of how many calories they need each day or the calorie content of foods and beverages they consume (USDA, 2010). That is not surprising given that the dietary energy content of food is not always obvious. Just one medium-size bran muffin can provide more than one-quarter of total calories for a woman who has a dietary goal of 1,200 calories per day. While dieters can estimate calorie content of foods using online databases, food labels, restaurant nutrition information sheets, and handbooks of nutrient information, it can be a tedious and confusing exercise. Consumers may look for ready-made food patterns and simple dietary guidelines as alternatives that can help with weight management.

Dietary Recommendations for Weight Management

The National Heart, Lung, and Blood Institute issued the first evidence-based guidelines for the treatment of adult obesity in 1998. Other groups, including the US Preventive Services Task Force in 2003, the American College of Physicians in 2005, and the American Dietetic Association in 2009, have formulated guidelines for weight-loss interventions and treatment.

Every five years, the US Department of Health and Human Services (DHHS) and US Department of Agriculture (USDA) jointly publish the Dietary Guidelines for Americans (DGA) based on the latest scientific evidence. A recent version was released in January 2010. The 2010 DGA define a healthy eating plan as one that:

- Emphasizes fruits, vegetables, whole grains, and fat-free or low-fat milk and milk products.

- Includes lean meats, poultry, fish, beans, eggs, and nuts.
- Is low in saturated fats, trans fats, cholesterol, salt, and added sugars.
- Stays within individual calorie needs.

The DGA are not specifically for weight loss as they are intended as an integrated set of messages to achieve an overall healthy eating pattern. However, they are presented as a range of recommended calorie intakes and food patterns based on an individual's age, sex, and activity level (USDA, 2010). Consumer-friendly advice and tools that apply to the 2010 DGA are also available. The website ChooseMyPlate.gov features links that allow consumers to:

- Look up a food.
- Get a personalized plan.
- Get weight-loss information.
- Analyze a diet.
- Ask a question.

Along with updated food patterns for the 2010 DGA a new graphic, MyPlate, was introduced in 2011 to replace the Food Guide Pyramid (FGP). Nutritionists often criticized the FGP, which was first promoted in 1992, for being misleading or hard to understand. The MyPlate graphic shown in **Figure 5.1** illustrates five food groups—fruits, vegetables, grains, protein, and dairy foods—using a familiar mealtime visual, a place setting.

Compared with the FGP, the MyPlate plan should be easier to apply because there is no need to figure out serving sizes of various foods. The new graphic is intended to be a reminder for healthy eating as it shows what a healthy plate should resemble. MyPlate will be used in an ongoing campaign to communicate essential dietary guidelines to consumers. For consumers who seek more information, or individualized guidance, the ChooseMyPlate.gov website elaborates on nutrition goals reflected in the plate's design. All the messages are based on the content of the 2010 DGA. The messages that are helpful for weight management include:

- Enjoy your food, but eat less.
- Avoid oversized portions.
- Make half your plate fruits and vegetables.
- Switch to fat-free or low-fat (1%) milk.
- Drink water instead of sugary drinks.

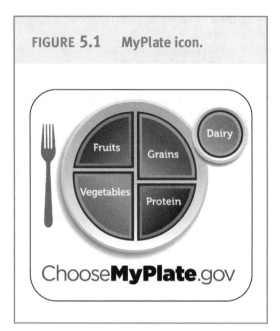

FIGURE **5.1** MyPlate icon.

Courtesy of: USDA.

Food Groups and Energy Density

The USDA MyPlate is based on a suggested ratio of food groups. Dietary messages based on this particular ratio can support general health as well as weight management.

Fruits and Vegetables Food Group

Professional weight management experts often use the USDA Guidelines in combination with other general strategies to reduce calorie intake. Common advice is to replace high-calorie foods with foods and beverages that are relatively lower in calories. The MyPlate message to "Make half your plate fruits and vegetables" may help individuals control total calorie intake and manage body weight because most fruits and vegetables are naturally low in fat and calories and they are filling. The property of foods being filling or satisfying is the key to understanding why fruits and vegetables can help in a weight management program. Research shows that, on a day-to-day basis, most individuals eat a fairly consistent weight of food regardless of the energy content. The volume of food people eat at a meal is what makes them feel full and stop eating (Ello-Martin, 2007). Water and fiber components increase the volume of foods and reduce energy density. **Energy density** is the number of calories in food relative to its weight. Foods with high calories in relation to their weight, such as fats and oils, are high-energy-dense foods. Fresh fruits and vegetables are low-energy-dense foods with few calories in relation to their weight. Energy density affects the total number of calories individuals consume. For the same number of calories a greater volume of low-energy-dense foods can be eaten compared to foods with high energy density. In this way, substituting fruits and vegetables for higher-calorie foods can help adults and children achieve and maintain a healthy weight.

Observational studies among adults have shown that lower-energy-dense diets are associated with lower overall energy intakes. The diets of normal-weight adults are lower in energy density than the diets of obese adults and higher-energy-dense diets are associated with higher BMI values (Ledikwe, 2006; Kral, 2004). In a five-day study where participants ate as much as they wanted from menus that alternated from low-energy-dense to high-energy-dense foods, the participants said they felt as full on 1,570 calories from the low-energy-dense diet as they did on a 3,000-calorie high-energy-dense diet (Duncan, 1983). Other research has shown that satiety is enhanced and meal energy intake is reduced when a large portion of a low-energy-dense food such as soup or salad is consumed at the start of the meal (Rolls, 2004; Flood, 2007). Long-term studies show that moderate weight loss was three times greater for people who ate low-energy-dense foods compared with those who followed a low-fat foods diet (Yao, 2001). Weight control is not the only benefit of eating more fruits and vegetables. Diets rich in fruits and vegetables may reduce the risk of some types of cancer and other chronic diseases. They also provide essential vitamins and minerals, fiber, and other components that contribute to good health.

Grains Food Group

A key consumer message, "Make at least half your grains whole grains," may also benefit weight management. Adding fruits, vegetables, and whole grains can dilute the calorie density of menu items. For example, extra vegetables and whole-grain bread will reduce the energy density of a meat sandwich. Fiber adds volume and provides a feeling of fullness so fewer overall calories may be consumed. Fiber is an important dietary component found only in plants, particularly vegetables, fruits, whole grains, nuts, and legumes. It does not provide much dietary energy as it is not digested in the small intestine but passes through to the colon where it may be partially metabolized by intestinal bacteria or eliminated as part of feces. Depending on the type of fiber, the calorie contribution ranges from 0 to 2 cal/g. The average American consumes about 15 g of fiber daily, well below the recommended levels of 25 g for women and 38 g for men (USDA, 2010).

USDA reports show that most of the grains consumed in the United States are refined grains such as white flour or white rice rather than whole grains. Whole grains consist of the entire grain kernel that contains the bran, germ, and endosperm. Examples include whole-wheat flour and brown rice. Refined grains have been milled to remove the bran and germ. This is done to give grains a fine texture and improve shelf life. Milling also removes dietary fiber, iron, and B vitamins. The MyPlate website provides details about types of whole grains and how the amount of fiber varies in whole grains versus refined grains.

Whole-grain intake is associated with a lower body weight (O'Neil, 2010). In a study of intake of dietary fiber, grain products, and weight gain in a cohort of nearly 75,000 women, weight gain was inversely associated with intake of high-fiber, whole-grain foods but positively related to the intake of refined-grain foods (Liu, 2003). Dietary fiber, regardless of the source, has also been linked to weight regulation. A review summarizing the effects of higher- versus lower-fiber diet interventions found that an increase of 14 g of fiber a day was associated with an average weight loss of 1.9 kg (4.2 lb) over about 4 months (Howarth, 2001). These analyses highlight the importance of fiber-rich foods such as fruits and vegetables for weight regulation.

Dairy Food Group

Another key consumer message is "Switch to fat-free or low-fat (one-percent) milk." The DGA suggests that everyone should include milk or calcium-fortified beverages at daily meals. Analyses in 2008 and 2009 showed a neutral association of the dairy food group with weight management, and limited short-term studies of dairy foods and weight change had inconsistent results (Lanou, 2008; Dove, 2009). It is also possible that confounding factors are linked with yogurt consumption. For example, people who eat yogurt may practice other health behaviors that influence their weight. Although a later review did find that yogurt consumption was associated with lower weight (Mozaffarian, 2011), mechanisms for the yogurt/weight relationship are unclear. However, a growing body of intriguing research suggests that intestinal bacteria, enhanced by the yogurt cultures, may influence energy harvesting and utilization (Duncan, 2008).

Protein Food Group

There is currently no research that suggests an independent relationship between long-term body weight and intake of the protein foods group (meat, poultry, seafood, beans and peas, eggs, processed soy products, nuts, and seeds). These foods are important sources of essential nutrients and should be part of any healthful diet (USDA, 2010).

Solid Fats and Added Sugars

Many popular foods and beverages contain "empty calories." These are foods that provide calories but

---

BOX 5.1 Solid Fats and Added Sugars

Solid fats are fats that are solid at room temperature, like butter, beef fat, and shortening. Solid fats may occur naturally in foods or they can be added when foods are processed or prepared.

Added sugars in typical American diets are sugars and syrups added to foods during processing, preparation, or at the table.

Data from: USDA Center for Nutrition Policy and Promotion.

few or no nutrients. Solid fats and added sugars (the USDA identifies these foods by the acronym SoFAS) are in the empty calorie category. Together, they comprise more than a third of the calories consumed by average Americans (USDA, 2010).

The SoFAS can make foods or beverages tasty and more appealing. They also add extra calories. While foods containing SoFAS are no more likely to contribute to weight gain than any other source of calories as long as total calories are within limits, as the amount of dietary energy from SoFAS increases, it becomes more difficult to stay within those limits. For most people, no more than about 5 to 15% of calories from SoFAS can be realistically accommodated in calorie-specific USDA Food Patterns.

One of the key recommendations of the DGA is "Choose and prepare foods and beverages with little added sugars or caloric sweeteners." Added sugars alone contribute an average of 16% of the total calories in American diets. As shown in **Figure 5.2**, the major sources of those added sugars are soda, energy drinks, and sports drinks, grain-based desserts, sugar-sweetened fruit drinks, dairy-based desserts, and candy (USDA, 2010).

It has been suggested that sugar-sweetened beverages (SSBs) are a significant contributor to the obesity epidemic, particularly for children and adolescents. Evidence indicates that consumption of SSBs in youth predicts weight gain in adulthood (Malik, 2010). It is thought that SSBs contribute to weight gain because of their

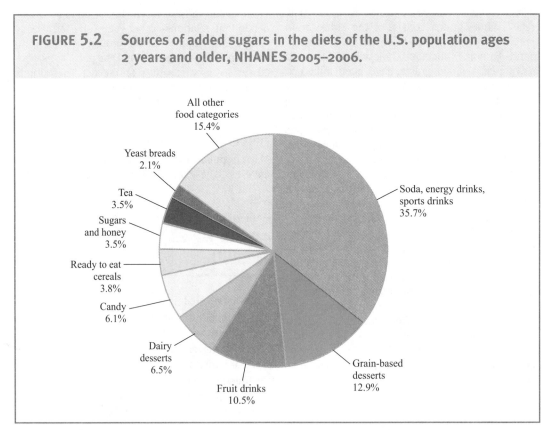

FIGURE 5.2   **Sources of added sugars in the diets of the U.S. population ages 2 years and older, NHANES 2005–2006.**

All other food categories 15.4%

Yeast breads 2.1%

Tea 3.5%

Sugars and honey 3.5%

Ready to eat cereals 3.8%

Candy 6.1%

Dairy desserts 6.5%

Fruit drinks 10.5%

Soda, energy drinks, sports drinks 35.7%

Grain-based desserts 12.9%

Reproduced from: U.S. Department of Agriculture and U.S. Department of Health and Human Services. Dietary Guidelines for Americans, 2010. 7th Edition, Washington, DC: U.S. Government Printing Office, December 2010, p. 29. *Data from*: National Cancer Institute. Sources of added sugars in the diets of the U.S. population ages 2 years and older, NHANES 2005–2006. Risk Factor Monitoring and Methods. Cancer Control and Population Sciences.

high-energy content, low satiety, and the view that liquid calories may not affect satiety to the extent required to suppress subsequent intake of solid foods (DiMeglio, 2000).

As sweetened beverages are the highest contributor to added sugar intake another DGA tip is "Drink water instead of sugary drinks." Details about added sugars and a chart that shows calories in soft drinks can be found on the discretionary calories page of the MyPlate.gov website. Energy intake in schoolchildren was shown to be significantly lower in water drinkers compared to non–water drinkers. One year of drinking only water was linked with a 31% reduction in the risk of being overweight (Malik, 2010).

Alcoholic Beverages

Reducing alcohol intake is an additional strategy to consume fewer calories. Alcohol contributes 7 cal/g and because alcohol is often consumed in mixtures with other beverages, the number of calories in an alcoholic drink can vary considerably. The relationship between alcohol use and weight

---

BOX 5.2 **Description of a Standard Alcoholic Drink**

A standard drink is about 14 g (0.6 oz) of pure alcohol.
Typically, this amount of alcohol is found in

- 12 oz of regular beer
- 8 oz of malt liquor
- 5 oz of wine
- 1.5 oz or a "shot" of 80-proof distilled spirits or liquor (e.g., gin, rum, vodka, or whiskey)

Source: CDC. Centers for Disease Control and Prevention. Alcohol and Public Health. 2011; http://www.cdc.gov/alcohol/faqs.htm#standDrink. Accessed July 20, 2011.

---

change is complex and research findings have been inconsistent. Moderate alcohol consumption (no more than one drink per day for women and no more than two drinks per day for men) is not significantly related to weight gain. However, more than moderate consumption of alcohol over time is associated with increased weight (USDA, 2010). In an analysis of alcohol consumption in relation to weight change in women over a period of 8 years, the smallest weight gain was seen among women who were moderate drinkers (Wannamethee, 2004). Further analyses are needed to assess the effects of sex, beverage type, and amount of intake on the alcohol and weight relationship.

Portion Control

The following is dietary portion control advice from the DGA:

- Enjoy your food, but eat less.
- Avoid oversized portions.

Even the most healthful foods may cause weight gain if sizeable portions provide excess energy. When choosing appropriate amounts of food the difference between a portion and a serving can be confusing. Serving size is a standardized unit of measuring foods—for example, a cup or ounce—used in the DGA and listed on a product's Nutrition Facts label. A portion is the amount of a food served in a single eating occasion, such as a meal or a snack. It is what is offered to a person in a restaurant, the quantity a person chooses to put on a dinner plate, or the amount in a typical package of ready-to-eat foods. A portion and a serving size may be equal, but frequently they are different. For example, bagels or muffins are often sold in portion sizes that are at least two servings. The new USDA MyPlate does not describe foods in terms of servings. Food group recommendations are made in household units: cups for fruits, vegetables, and dairy (milk and soymilk) and ounce equivalents for grains and protein foods.

To learn how much to eat each day from the five food groups for weight management, individuals can create a customized Daily Food Plan (see **Figure 5.3**) on the USDA website by entering age, sex, height, weight, and activity level. The

FIGURE 5.3 My Daily Food Plan.

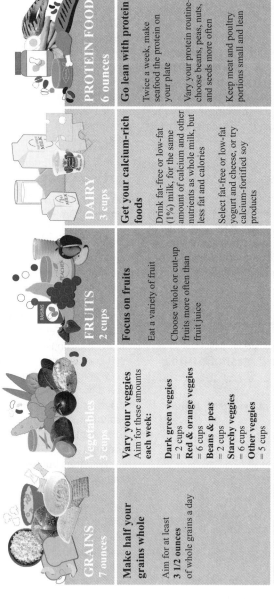

My Daily Food Plan

Based on the information you provided, this is your daily recommended amount for each food group.

GRAINS 7 ounces	Vegetables 3 cups	FRUITS 2 cups	DAIRY 3 cups	PROTEIN FOODS 6 ounces
Make half your grains whole	**Vary your veggies** Aim for these amounts each week:	**Focus on fruits**	**Get your calcium-rich foods**	**Go lean with protein**
Aim for at least **3 1/2 ounces** of whole grains a day	**Dark green veggies** = 2 cups **Red & orange veggies** = 6 cups **Beans & peas** = 2 cups **Starchy veggies** = 6 cups **Other veggies** = 5 cups	Eat a variety of fruit Choose whole or cut-up fruits more often than fruit juice	Drink fat-free or low-fat (1%) milk, for the same amount of calcium and other nutrients as whole milk, but less fat and calories Select fat-free or low-fat yogurt and cheese, or try calcium-fortified soy products	Twice a week, make seafood the protein on your plate Vary your protein routine— choose beans, peas, nuts, and seeds more often Keep meat and poultry portions small and lean

Find your balance between food and physical activity

Be physically active for at least 150 minutes each week

Your results are based on a 2200 calorie pattern.

Know your limits on fats, sugars, and sodium

Your allowance for oils is **6 teaspoons** a day.
Limit calories from solid fats and added sugars to **270 calories** a day.
Reduce sodium intake to less than **2300 mg** a day.

Name: _____

This calorie level is only an estimate of your needs. Monitor your body weight to see if you need to adjust your calorie intake plan allows a choice of calorie options designed to gradually achieve a healthy weight. There are also worksheets to track daily progress.

Even without scales or cups, it is possible to eat all types of foods in moderation at home or when eating out. Appropriate food portions can be visualized by comparison to objects of similar size. For example, 3 oz of meat or poultry is about the size of a deck of cards. One-half cup of cooked pasta or potato is similar in volume to half of a tennis ball or what could fit in an adult's cupped hand. More examples of how to judge the amount of foods can be downloaded at the NHLBI Portion Distortion website listed in the Resources section of this chapter.

Numerous studies have shown that people will eat more when they are offered larger portions. In a study of sandwich size and food consumption women consumed 31% more energy and men consumed 56% more energy when they were served a 12-in. sandwich compared to a 6-in. sandwich. Reports of hunger and fullness did not differ significantly whether subjects consumed an 8-in., 10-in., or 12-in. sandwich. Subjects who ate more food reported feeling fuller, but they did not compensate for the extra calories at the subsequent meal (Ledikwe, 2005). In the "popcorn test" people given large containers of popcorn ate an average of 44% more (equal to about 120 kcal) than those who got small containers, even though the popcorn was stale (Wansink, 2005). When consumers regularly eat large amounts they get a distorted impression of what a reasonable portion size really is. Large food portions even affect children's energy intake at meals. Children ranging in age between 2 and 9 years were given either an age-appropriate entrée or a portion twice as large as the age-appropriate portion. Children as young as 2 years old had a 13% higher energy intake at the meal when given the larger entrée than when a smaller portion was provided. Children took a similar number of bites regardless of the portion size, but they took bigger bites when they were served a larger portion (Fisher, 2007).

There is a positive association between the frequency of eating out in restaurants or fast food outlets and increased body weight. This may be due to greater portion sizes and/or higher energy density. Those who often eat fast food have significantly higher odds of being overweight compared with those who do not regularly consume fast food. Analysis of a 15-year study of adults revealed that eating fast food three times per week is associated with a 1.6 to 2.2 kg (3.5 to 4.8 lb) weight gain (Pereira, 2005).

Food Labels

The Nutrition Facts label is intended to be easy-to-use information that allows purchasers to understand the nutritional value of a food, compare products, and increase or decrease consumption of nutrients or calories. Food labels also can help people understand the relative size of food portions. For example, one serving of potato chips might supply 100 calories. When the serving size is only 10 chips and there are 10 servings per bag, the calories add up if a person finishes the entire contents. The Nutrition Facts labels on beverage containers often give the calories for only part of the contents. The label on a 20-oz bottle may list the number of calories in 8 oz even though the bottle contains 20 oz or 2.5 servings. Details about reading food labels to help with weight management can be found online in the USDA Guidelines Appendix 4; the website is listed in the Resources section of this chapter.

Nutrition and health professionals have consistently called for calorie and other nutrition information to be prominent in restaurants and other venues where food is purchased. In a provision of the 2010 healthcare reform law, restaurants, convenience stores, concession stands, and vending machines would have to display calorie information for the food products they sell. Under the regulations, any restaurant with 20 or more locations, including table-service establishments, fast food outlets, bakeries, and coffee shops, would have to disclose calories "clearly and prominently" on menus or menu boards, including drive-through order stations by 2012. Other nutritional information, such as sodium and fat content, would have to be available upon request (FDA, 2011). Even before that law was to go into effect, menu labeling laws were passed in dozens of states and localities. Food industry groups anticipated the rules and some restaurant chains voluntarily began to provide the information in stores and on websites.

Timing of Meals

Nutritionists usually advise eating small, frequent meals as a good strategy for weight loss. This idea was based on a body of research showing an inverse relationship between meal frequency and BMI. Many studies found that people who reported eating more times per day were less likely to be overweight. Eating breakfast, in particular, was recommended because routinely eating a healthy breakfast was associated with energy balance and weight control (Cho, 2003). Data showed that obesity was associated with skipping breakfast four or more times a week. However, it was only low-energy breakfasts that were associated with lower BMI and lower energy intake. A high-energy breakfast consisting of high-fat dairy, meat, and/or eggs could have a more negative effect on weight and cardiovascular health than not eating breakfast at all (Greenwood, 2008).

The assumption that the more times per day people ate, the less likely they were to be overweight was challenged in a 2011 report by McCrory and colleagues (2011). Studies that found the apparent inverse relationship between meal frequency and body weight were based on self-reported intake. It has been shown that people who weigh more generally tend to underreport their food intake. When underreporting is taken into account in studies on eating frequency and body weight, the results generally showed that it was actually the leaner people who eat less often while overweight and obese people eat more often during a day. The few intervention studies on eating frequency show no significant effect of eating frequency on body weight. An American Dietetic Association position paper states that, as research does not support absolute meal frequency or breakfast recommendations for weight management, the current appropriate recommendation is that total caloric intake should be distributed throughout the day and should include breakfast (Seagle, 2009).

Specific Diet Plans

Calorie-Reduced Diets

The NHLBI 1998 obesity guidelines panel reviewed reports of the effectiveness of numerous diets on weight loss. The composite results of the trials indicated that a low-calorie diet (LCD) containing 800 to 1,500 kcal/day consumed as liquid formula, nutritional bars, conventional food, or a combination of these items would produce about an 8% weight loss after 16 to 26 weeks of treatment (NHLBI, 1998). Based on strong evidence, the panel recommended that LCDs be advised for weight loss in overweight and obese persons. The specific recommendation was: A diet that is individually planned to help create a deficit of 500 to 1,000 cal/day should be an integral part of any program aimed at achieving a weight loss of 1 to 2 lb per week (NHLBI, 1998). Application of that advice could be based on a variety of energy reduction strategies such as those that focus on calorie counting, energy density, particular macronutrient composition, portion-controlled meals, or general healthful eating.

Recommended Macronutrient Distribution

Even though total calorie intake is the vital issue for weight management, it is important to consider essential nutrients and other healthful aspects of food and beverages when devising an eating pattern. Carbohydrates, protein, and fat are the main sources of calories in the diet and most foods and beverages contain combinations of these macronutrients. The Food and Nutrition Board of the Institute of Medicine has established ranges for the percentage of calories in the diet that come from these sources. These ratios, associated with reduced risk for chronic diseases, while providing essential nutrients, are defined as the Acceptable Macronutrient Distribution Range (AMDR). The AMDRs for adults as a percentage of calories are:

- Protein: 10–35%
- Fat: 20–35%
- Carbohydrate: 45–65%

There is a good deal of controversy about whether particular macronutrients differentially affect satiety, diet adherence, and other factors that would affect energy balance (Astrup, 2008). Many popular diets focus on the effects of individual macronutrients as components that can make weight management easier or more effective.

Low-Fat, High-Carbohydrate, High-Fiber Diets

Low-fat, high-carbohydrate, high-fiber diets such as those proposed by Dean Ornish and Nathan Pritikin emphasize whole grains, fruits, vegetables, and low-fat protein while reducing fat to as low as 10% of total daily calories. These diets limit all types of dietary fat including saturated, trans, monounsaturated, and polyunsaturated fats. Dietary fat alone does not necessarily cause excess weight gain, but fat is a concentrated source of calories. It has 9 cal/g whereas protein and carbohydrates only have 4 cal/g. In a given weight of food the most efficient way to reduce calories is to cut back on the fat. The NHLBI guidelines suggest limiting total fat to 30% or less of total calories. For a 2,000 calorie diet that would mean about 660 fat calories, or 75 g of fat in meals each day. Studies show that people consume more total energy with high-fat diets compared with low-fat diets (NHLBI, 1998). Nevertheless, reducing the percentage of dietary fat alone will not produce weight loss unless total calories are also reduced (NHLBI, 1998).

For optimal health, the carbohydrates in low-fat diets should come mainly from naturally occurring complex carbohydrates, such as those found in whole grains, beans and peas, vegetables, and fruits, while refined grains and foods with added sugars should be limited. Strong positive associations with weight increase are seen with diets high in starches, refined grains, and processed foods (Ledikwe, 2007). As compared with less-processed, higher-fiber foods, it may be that starches and refined grains produce less satiety, so subsequent hunger signals occur sooner and total caloric intake could be increased (Bornet, 2007).

High-Protein, Low-Carbohydrate Diets

Diet plans such as Atkins, Zone, and South Beach are based on protein content that makes up 30 to 40% of the calories while carbohydrates are moderately or severely reduced. Carbohydrate monitoring may be based on the **glycemic index (GI)**. The GI assigns a number to foods depending on the speed at which carbohydrates are absorbed into circulation as glucose and the resulting effects on blood glucose levels. Foods with a higher value are digested quickly and create a quick rise in glucose and insulin levels whereas foods with a lower GI take longer to process, are absorbed more slowly, and theoretically keep the dieter feeling fuller longer. Because blood glucose response is affected by both the quality (glycemic index) and the quantity of carbohydrates in a meal, the **glycemic load** concept was developed. The glycemic load is calculated by multiplying the glycemic index of individual foods by the total amount of carbohydrates consumed.

The restriction of digestible carbohydrates that impact blood glucose is intended to switch metabolism from burning glucose as fuel to metabolizing stored body fat. There are a variety of food choices that can be used to make a plan that reduces carbohydrates and increases protein. The most healthful plans would replace high-carbohydrate starches and sugars from soft drinks and refined grains with lean animal protein, plant protein, and lower fat dairy products, without reducing fruits, vegetables, and whole grains. If dietary fats are increased, they should be monounsaturated and polyunsaturated, such as those found in seafood, nuts, seeds, and oils.

There are reports that high-protein, low-carbohydrate food plans are more satisfying than low-fat diets. Several short-term studies suggest that, despite equal energy intakes, initial weight loss during the first 4 weeks is greater with a low-carbohydrate diet than with high-carbohydrate diets (Westman, 2002). In a research study at Stanford University premenopausal overweight or obese women on the Atkins diet lost significantly more weight at 12 months compared with participants who followed low-fat or traditional diets (Gardner, 2007).

Medically Supervised Very-Low-Calorie Diets

Medically supervised clinic-based and proprietary programs such as Optifast and Medifast place patients on very-low-calorie-diet (VLCD) plans that are usually about 800 calories per day. Liquid diets and nutrition bars replace ordinary food. The theory is that a VLCD could be an effective method for obese individuals to lose weight quickly if they have the medical supervision critical for following it safely. After initial weight loss, a slow reintroduction to conventional foods and education about new ways of healthy eating is intended to promote long-term success. Patients completing these programs can lose approximately 15 to 25% of their initial weight during 3 to 6 months of treatment and maintain a loss of 8 to 9% at 1 year (Tsai, 2005). However, the success rate might be overestimated given that the many reports did not include people who dropped out of the study. Several randomized trials have indicated that 1 year after the diet is completed VLCDs do not result in any greater weight reduction when compared to other, less stringent, diets. In fact, in women weight regain was greater after VLCD than LCD therapy (Torgerson, 1997; Jones, 2007).

Research Comparison of Diets

Hundreds of both complicated and simple diet plans have been promoted as the best way to lose weight, but currently there is no scientific evidence to show that any one diet or proportion of foods or macronutrients is more effective than another in the long run. **Table 5.2** describes some of the most common diet plans including potential benefits and disadvantages. A randomized trial comparing various diets that restricted carbohydrates, limited fats, increased protein, and/or limited calories showed that each diet was moderately effective for reducing weight at 1 year. The authors concluded that adherence to any eating plan that restricts calorie intake can lead to successful weight loss (Dansinger, 2007). In a 2-year study weight loss was similar among diets that had different ratios of fat, carbohydrates, and protein. Satiety, hunger, and satisfaction with the diets were also similar among all groups. Any possible effect of the macronutrient differences may have been diluted because study participants may had difficulty maintaining their assigned macronutrient ratios for the duration of the study and only about 15% of participants managed at least 10% weight loss (Sacks, 2009). Scientific

assessment of weight-loss diets indicates that it is adherence to a diet, not the diet itself, that makes the difference.

Popular Diet Plans

Adherence to a diet may be increased by group support or structured meal plans. For individuals who like the structure and support of a group, there is a wide variety of weight-loss options. Self-help groups such as Overeaters Anonymous (OA) and Take Off Pounds Sensibly (TOPS) are free of charge and are led by group members. TOPS members work with a physician to develop a personal food plan. Participants maintain accountability through private weekly weigh-ins, and they receive ongoing group support. OA addresses problems associated with compulsive eating and encourages members to abstain from foods that might act as triggers to overeat. The OA philosophy guides participants to physical, emotional, and spiritual health. There is minimal scientific evidence available to judge success rates from these two groups.

Commercial franchises such WeightWatchers, Jenny Craig, and Nutrisystem rely on counselors to provide services to clients. The counselors are often individuals who have been on the program and have successfully lost weight and maintained that weight loss. The programs offer support meetings, materials, and even beverages, nutrition bars, and easy-to-prepare meals. When individuals are given a fixed amount of food with known calorie content, mealtime choices are simplified. Several studies have shown that commercially packaged meals, controlled for portion size and energy content, help consumers lose weight. In addition, drop-out rates are lower for meal replacement plans than for conventional diets (Ello-Martin, 2005).

Most support groups have websites that offer meal plans, recipes, chats with other dieters, and e-mail advice from experts, such as dietitians and psychologists. Internet-based information and social networking can be used on its own or it may be a useful supplement to other programs. The convenience of online record keeping of daily food intake, physical activity, and weight changes could possibly increase adherence to a program.

TABLE 5.2   Comparison of Common Diet Plans for Weight Management

Diet plan	Description and/or commercial examples	Claims/advantages	Disadvantages
Very-low-calorie diet	Provides 200–800 kcal/day **Examples:** Optifast, Medifast	Rapid weight loss No concern about meal planning and appropriate food choices	Not nutritionally adequate Requires medical supervision and frequent follow-up Long-term weight loss does not differ from low-calorie diets
Calorie reduction diet	500–1,000 kcal/day deficit Usually based on Acceptable Macronutrient Distribution Ranges (AMDR) **Examples:** Most typical weight-loss diets	Possible weight loss of 1–2 lb/week Can be used for long-term weight management Can include most foods	Calorie counting is usually necessary Slow rate of weight loss may be discouraging
Low-fat, high-carbohydrate, calorie controlled	Fat intake less than 20% of total energy **Examples:** WeightWatchers, Volumetrics, Pritikin, Ornish (no more than 10% calories from fat)	May efficiently reduce total calorie intake Generally nutritionally balanced, does not exclude major food groups Suitable for vegetarians Fits with most lifestyles Support groups offer encouragement	Effective only if total energy intake is also reduced Decreased long-term compliance due to many food restrictions Expensive weekly meetings with some groups
High-protein, high-fat, low carbohydrates	Diets may be accomplished in phases: induction, ongoing weight loss, premaintenance, and lifetime maintenance **Examples:** South Beach (initial stage), Atkins (20 g of carbohydrate daily for 2 to 3 months, 50 g daily thereafter)	Quick initial weight loss No measuring No hunger Unlimited protein-rich and fatty foods	Intake of carbohydrates and calories is extremely low The eating regimen is very restricted Low in many valuable nutrients Constipation may also occur as a consequence of avoiding typically high-fiber foods Not suited for vegetarians

(continues)

TABLE 5.2   Comparison of Common Diet Plans for Weight Management (continued)

Diet plan	Description and/or commercial examples	Claims/advantages	Disadvantages
High-protein, moderate fat, moderate carbohydrates	Proteins encouraged and some types of carbohydrates limited but not restricted **Example:** Zone Diet (40-30-30 ratio of carbohydrates to protein to fat)	Promotes use of fat for energy Supports healthful eating habits such as portion control and sugar reduction Allows for ample fruits and vegetables	Carbohydrate recommendations lack whole grains, low in fiber May be complex, confusing, and time-consuming to plan meals
	Example: South Beach Diet (later stages) Replaces "bad carbs" and "bad fats" with "good carbs" and "good fats" Done in three phases, each progressively becoming more liberal	Fairly balanced after the initial strict phase Does not rely on high levels of saturated fat No calorie or fat counting Encourages regular meals and snacks	May be expensive
Meal replacements	Meal replacement diets provide between 800 and 1,000 cal/day The dieter is instructed to replace two meals a day with meal replacement products (shakes, soups, bars, cookies, and drinks) The dieter is then encouraged to eat a portion-controlled, healthy dinner **Examples:** Jenny Craig, Nutrisystem, WeightWatchers meal plan	Portion-controlled No meal preparation Minimal dealing with food Quick initial weight loss Prepackaged frozen meals are convenient and offer many options	The products can be expensive Many gain weight back when stop using products

There are hundreds of other diet plans and many have very specific recommendations that make them unique; however, diet composition is generally based on low-calorie, low-fat, or low-carbohydrate patterns.

How Do We Know What Works?

To determine what diets work best in real life scientists study individuals who have lost weight and actually kept it off. The National Weight Control Registry (NWCR) is a database of nearly 3,000 individuals who have been recognized as being successful at long-term weight maintenance. Ninety-eight percent of NWCR participants report that they modified their food intake in some way to lose weight. However, researchers who investigated the characteristics of these individuals could not identify any single diet or food plan common to registry members. Some participants reported that they restricted their intake of certain foods; others counted calories or grams of fat, or used liquid formulas. Only a minority followed a low-carbohydrate diet. Many stated that, while they were conscious of food quantity, they did not deprive themselves of favorite high-calorie foods as they would if they were just waiting for the end of a dieting regimen. While some individuals participated in formal weight-loss programs or groups, most devised personalized weight-loss and maintenance plans using ideas from their own earlier experiences (Phelan, 2006). The data from NWCR research support the view that a wide variety of diet strategies can be effective. The diet associated with the highest success is one that an individual enjoys and is most likely to adhere to over time.

Summary

Matching dietary energy intake with energy expenditure is essential to weight management. The appropriate calorie intake a person needs each day varies depending on age, sex, height, weight, and physical activity. Information about calorie needs can be gathered from tables of general estimates or individual requirements can be calculated with online tools such as those available on the USDA Dietary Guidelines website. The most uncomplicated way to assess an individual's appropriate calorie needs is to monitor body weight. Calorie intake can be increased or decreased in response to weight changes over time. Energy consumption from foods and beverages is influenced by such factors as patterns of eating, levels of satiety or fullness, or portion sizes. A scientifically based healthy eating pattern that addresses these issues is offered through the Dietary Guidelines for Americans (DGA). The latest version was released in January 2010. The DGA are not specifically geared toward weight loss; however, they may be a basis for choosing food patterns for weight management. The MyPlate messages are helpful for reducing energy intake as they provide guidelines for choosing lower-energy-dense foods. There are numerous dietary options for inducing weight loss, and popular diets vary dramatically in their macronutrient composition. Research studies show that no one diet plan or specific macronutrient distribution works equally well to reduce calories for everyone. Because most people who try to lose weight by dieting do not manage to keep off the weight in the long run one of the keys to successful weight control is finding a reduced-calorie eating plan that the individual likes and can adhere to long term.

Because of this lack of long-term weight-loss maintenance, health professionals are shifting their focus from trying to identify the best weight-loss diet to understanding a broader range of behaviors and characteristics of those who lose weight successfully and those who do not.

Critical Thinking Questions

Question: "Easily lose as much weight as you wish without wasting a minute of your day at http://www.get-slim-while-you-sleep.com/"

Advertisements such as these that sell miracle products or schemes that promise easy, fast weight loss without the need to give up favorite foods or increase physical activity flood the marketplace. Locate and critique several examples of these types of advertisements.

Question: More of the foods that we eat at home tend to be eaten out of a bag or package rather than from a plate. How does this statement affect application of the MyPlate concept for promoting healthy eating?

Resources

American Dietetic Association Resources
www.eatright.org
Eat More, Weigh Less?
http://www.cdc.gov/healthyweight/healthy_eating/energy_density.html
Self Nutrition Data: Know What You Eat
http://nutritiondata.self.com/
How to Understand and Use the Nutrition Facts Label
http://www.fda.gov/Food/ResourcesForYou/Consumers/NFLPM/ucm274593.htm
How to Use Fruits and Vegetables to Help Manage Your Weight
http://www.cdc.gov/healthyweight/healthy_eating/fruits_vegetables.html
MyPlate
http://www.choosemyplate.gov/index.html
Portion Distortion
http://hp2010.nhlbihin.net/portion/keep.htm
Using the Food Label to Track Calories, Nutrients, and Ingredients (USDA Guidelines Appendix 4)
http://www.cnpp.usda.gov/Publications/DietaryGuidelines/2010/PolicyDoc/PolicyDoc.pdf
National Weight Control Registry
http://www.nwcr.ws/

References

Astrup A. Dietary management of obesity. *JPEN J Parenter Enteral Nutr.* Sep–Oct 2008;32(5):575–577.

Bornet FR, Jardy-Gennetier AE, Jacquet N, Stowell J. Glycaemic response to foods: impact on satiety and long-term weight regulation. *Appetite.* Nov 2007; 49(3):535–553.

CDC. Centers for Disease Control. Alcohol and Public Health. *CDC. 2010.* 2011; http://www.cdc.gov/alcohol/faqs.htm#standDrink. Accessed July 20, 2011.

Cho S, Dietrich M, Brown CJ, Clark CA, Block G. The effect of breakfast type on total daily energy intake and body mass index: results from the Third National Health and Nutrition Examination Survey (NHANES III). *J Am Coll Nutr.* Aug 2003;22(4):296–302.

Dansinger ML, Tatsioni A, Wong JB, Chung M, Balk EM. Meta-analysis: the effect of dietary counseling for weight loss. *Ann Intern Med.* Jul 3 2007;147(1): 41–50.

DiMeglio DP, Mattes RD. Liquid versus solid carbohydrate: effects on food intake and body weight. *Int J Obes Relat Metab Disord.* Jun 2000;24(6):794–800.

Dove ER, Hodgson JM, Puddey IB, Beilin LJ, Lee YP, Mori TA. Skim milk compared with a fruit drink acutely reduces appetite and energy intake in overweight men and women. *Am J Clin Nutr.* Jul 2009;90(1): 70–75.

Duncan KH, Bacon JA, Weinsier RL. The effects of high and low energy density diets on satiety, energy intake, and eating time of obese and nonobese subjects. *Am J Clin Nutr.* May 1983;37(5):763–767.

Duncan SH, Lobley GE, Holtrop G, et al. Human colonic microbiota associated with diet, obesity and weight loss. *Int J Obes (Lond).* Nov 2008;32(11):1720-1724.

Dunn CL, Hannan PJ, Jeffery RW, Sherwood NE, Pronk NP, Boyle R. The comparative and cumulative effects of a dietary restriction and exercise on weight loss. *Int J Obes (Lond).* Jan 2006;30(1):112–121.

Ello-Martin JA, Ledikwe JH, Rolls BJ. The influence of food portion size and energy density on energy intake: implications for weight management. *Am J Clin Nutr.* Jul 2005;82(1 Suppl):236S-241S.

FDA. Food and Drug Administration. Overview of FDA Proposed Labeling Requirements for Restaurants, Similar Retail Food Establishments and Vending Machines. 2011; http://www.fda.gov/Food/LabelingNutrition/ucm248732.htm. Accessed August 10, 2011.

Fisher JO, Liu Y, Birch LL, Rolls BJ. Effects of portion size and energy density on young children's intake at a meal. *Am J Clin Nutr.* Jul 2007;86(1):174–179.

Flood JE, Rolls BJ. Soup preloads in a variety of forms reduce meal energy intake. *Appetite.* Nov 2007; 49(3):626–634.

Gardner CD, Kiazand A, Alhassan S, et al. Comparison of the Atkins, Zone, Ornish, and LEARN diets for change in weight and related risk factors among overweight premenopausal women: the A TO Z Weight Loss Study: a randomized trial. *JAMA.* Mar 7 2007;297(9):969–977.

Greenwood JL, Stanford JB. Preventing or improving obesity by addressing specific eating patterns. *J Am Board Fam Med.* Mar–Apr 2008;21(2):135–140.

Howarth NC, Saltzman E, Roberts SB. Dietary fiber and weight regulation. *Nutr Rev.* May 2001;59(5): 129–139.

Jones LR, Wilson CI, Wadden TA. Lifestyle modification in the treatment of obesity: an educational challenge and opportunity. *Clin Pharmacol Ther.* May 2007;81(5):776–777.

Kral TV, Rolls BJ. Energy density and portion size: their independent and combined effects on energy intake. *Physiol Behav.* Aug 2004;82(1):131–138.

Lanou AJ, Barnard ND. Dairy and weight loss hypothesis: an evaluation of the clinical trials. *Nutr Rev.* May 2008;66(5):272–279.

Ledikwe JH, Blanck HM, Kettel Khan L, et al. Dietary energy density is associated with energy intake and weight status in US adults. *Am J Clin Nutr.* Jun 2006;83(6):1362–1368.

Ledikwe JH, Ello-Martin JA, Rolls BJ. Portion sizes and the obesity epidemic. *J Nutr.* Apr 2005;135(4):905–909.

Ledikwe JH, Rolls BJ, Smiciklas-Wright H, et al. Reductions in dietary energy density are associated with weight loss in overweight and obese participants in the PREMIER trial. *Am J Clin Nutr.* May 2007; 85(5):1212–1221.

Liu S, Willett WC, Manson JE, Hu FB, Rosner B, Colditz G. Relation between changes in intakes of dietary fiber and grain products and changes in weight and development of obesity among middle-aged women. *Am J Clin Nutr.* Nov 2003;78(5):920–927.

Malik VS, Popkin BM, Bray GA, Despres JP, Hu FB. Sugar-sweetened beverages, obesity, type 2 diabetes mellitus, and cardiovascular disease risk. *Circulation.* Mar 23 2010;121(11):1356–1364.

McCrory MA, Campbell WW. Effects of eating frequency, snacking, and breakfast skipping on energy regulation: symposium overview. *J Nutr.* Jan 2011;141(1): 144–147.

Mozaffarian D, Hao T, Rimm EB, Willett WC, Hu FB. Changes in diet and lifestyle and long-term weight gain in women and men. *N Engl J Med.* Jun 23 2011; 364(25):2392–2404.

NHLBI. National Heart, Lung, and Blood Institute. Clinical guidelines on the identification, evaluation, and treatment of overweight and obesity in adults: executive summary. Vol. No. 98-4083. Bethesda, MD: National Institutes of Health; 1998.

O'Neil CE, Zanovec M, Cho SS, Nicklas TA. Whole grain and fiber consumption are associated with lower body weight measures in US adults: National Health and Nutrition Examination Survey 1999–2004. *Nutr Res.* Dec 2010;30(12):815–822.

Pereira MA, Kartashov AI, Ebbeling CB, et al. Fast-food habits, weight gain, and insulin resistance (the CARDIA study): 15-year prospective analysis. *Lancet.* Jan 1–7 2005;365(9453):36–42.

Phelan S, Wyatt HR, Hill JO, Wing RR. Are the eating and exercise habits of successful weight losers changing? *Obesity (Silver Spring).* Apr 2006;14(4):710–716.

Rolls BJ, Roe LS, Meengs JS. Salad and satiety: energy density and portion size of a first-course salad affect energy intake at lunch. *J Am Diet Assoc.* Oct 2004;104(10):1570–1576.

Sacks FM, Bray GA, Carey VJ, et al. Comparison of weight-loss diets with different compositions of fat, protein, and carbohydrates. *N Engl J Med.* Feb 26 2009; 360(9):859–873.

Seagle HM, Strain GW, Makris A, Reeves RS. Position of the American Dietetic Association: weight management. *J Am Diet Assoc.* Feb 2009;109(2):330–346.

Torgerson JS, Lissner L, Lindroos AK, Kruijer H, Sjostrom L. VLCD plus dietary and behavioural support versus support alone in the treatment of severe obesity. A randomised two-year clinical trial. *Int J Obes Relat Metab Disord.* Nov 1997; 21(11):987–994.

Tsai AG, Wadden TA. Systematic review: an evaluation of major commercial weight loss programs in the

United States. *Ann Intern Med.* Jan 4 2005;142(1): 56-66.

USDA. *U.S. Department of Agriculture Dietary Guidelines for Americans, 2010.* 7th ed. Washington, DC: U.S. Government Printing Office; 2010.

Wannamethee SG, Field AE, Colditz GA, Rimm EB. Alcohol intake and 8-year weight gain in women: a prospective study. *Obes Res.* Sep 2004;12(9): 1386–1396.

Wansink B, Kim J. Bad popcorn in big buckets: portion size can influence intake as much as taste. *J Nutr Educ Behav.* Sep–Oct 2005;37(5):242–245.

Westman EC, Yancy WS, Edman JS, Tomlin KF, Perkins CE. Effect of 6-month adherence to a very low carbohydrate diet program. *Am J Med.* Jul 2002;113(1): 30–36.

Yao M, Roberts SB. Dietary energy density and weight regulation. *Nutr Rev.* Aug 2001;59(8 Pt 1):247–258.

CHAPTER 6

PHYSICAL ACTIVITY

READER OBJECTIVES

- Describe the role of physical activity in energy balance related to weight management
- Distinguish the difference between exercise and lifestyle physical activity
- Discuss how physical activity trends are influenced by demographic factors
- Differentiate between the amount and type of physical activity recommended for general health benefits, weight loss, and preventing weight regain
- Compare the role aerobic and strength-training types of physical activities have on weight loss and weight maintenance
- Describe how physical activity is related to metabolic health
- Review self-monitoring tools and websites for assessing and encouraging energy expenditure

CHAPTER OUTLINE

Energy Balance and Physical Activity

In addition to the multiple health benefits associated with **physical activity (PA)**, energy expenditure is an essential factor that determines whether an individual is able to maintain a healthy body weight, lose excess body weight, or sustain weight loss. A healthful body weight is dependent on maintaining a stable energy balance. To prevent weight gain, energy expenditure must match energy intake. To create a negative energy balance that results in weight loss, total energy expenditure (TEE) must exceed energy intake. Negative energy balance may be achieved either by increasing PA, or reducing food intake, or both. In several studies, prolonged low levels of PA were related to increased incidence of obesity (Wing, 2001; Elfhag, 2005). A study of more than 5,000 men and women showed that, after controlling for BMI, age, socioeconomic status, smoking, and comorbidities, inactive participants were more than twice as likely to gain weight over a 10-year period as the more active individuals (Haapanen, 1997). Increasing PA is a logical tool for prevention of obesity.

Definitions of Physical Activity

Two terms used to describe human movement are *physical activity* and *exercise*. While they are often used interchangeably, their definitions differ. The PA component of TEE is composed of all the ordinary activities of daily living such as standing, walking, and lifting and carrying, as well as purposeful activity. Purposeful activity or exercise can include brisk walking, dancing, lifting weights, climbing on playground equipment, or playing an active sport.

The amount of energy burned during PA is influenced by weight, exercise intensity, sex, and age. **Table 6.1** shows examples of the energy required per hour for various activities according to weight and exercise intensity. Numerous websites provide individualized estimates of kilocalories burned when weight, age, sex, and type of activity are entered into a calculator. See the websites

---

BOX 6.1   Definitions and Types of Physical Activity Adapted from 2008 Physical Activity Guidelines for Americans.

Physical activity: Any bodily movement produced by the contraction of skeletal muscle that increases energy expenditure above a basal level.

Inactivity: Not engaging in any regular pattern of PA beyond daily functioning.

Lifestyle activities: Examples include taking the stairs instead of using the elevator, walking to do errands instead of driving, or parking farther away than usual to walk to a destination.

Exercise: A type of PA that is planned, structured, and purposeful where improvement or maintenance of physical fitness is the objective. All exercise is PA, but not all PA is exercise.

MET or Metabolic Equivalent: *MET* is a term used to express the ratio of a person's metabolic rate while resting with their metabolic rate while performing a task. One MET is roughly the energy expenditure required to sit quietly and is measured as 1 kilocalorie per kilogram per hour (1 kcal/kg/hr).

Light-intensity activity: PA that is done at 1.1 to 2.9 METs.

Moderate-intensity physical activity: PA that is done at 3.0 to 5.9 METs.

Vigorous-intensity physical activity: PA that is done at 6.0 or more METs.

Data from: USDHHS. U.S. Department of Health and Human Services. 2008 Physical Activity Guidelines for Americans. Washington, D.C. http://www.health.gov/paguidelines/pdf/. Accessed August 2009.

TABLE 6.1 Kilocalories Burned per Hour According to Weight and Exercise Intensity

	125 lb	150 lb	200 lb
Bicycling, for leisure	175	190	225
Running, 12 min/mile	400	450	520
Walking, for leisure	145	160	190

Data from: Ainsworth BE, Haskell WL, Herrmann SD, Meckes N, Bassett DR Jr, Tudor-Locke C, Greer JL, Vezina J, Whitt-Glover MC, Leon AS. 2011 Compendium of physical activities: a second update of codes and MET values. *Med Sci Sports Exerc.* 2011;43(8):1575–1581.

listed in the Resources section of this chapter for more information.

Trends in Physical Activity

Despite the numerous benefits of PA associated with good health and longevity, over 50% of adults in the United States do not get enough. More than a quarter of Americans do not engage in any leisure-time PA such as running, walking, calisthenics, gardening, golf, or other sports (CDC, 2008). Daily activity is low due to numerous aspects of contemporary life. In many parts of the country, it is necessary to have a vehicle to navigate urban sprawl. The result is that less walking is required for moving about. Work-related PA has also decreased considerably as a result of the increasing use of labor-saving devices at work and at home. While each of these energy-saving efficiencies may reduce PA only slightly, they all add up to have an important impact on TEE.

According to Shape Up America! the amount of exercise necessary for the average American to maintain a healthy weight is estimated to be about 10,000 steps a day (Shape Up America, 2010). In contrast with those suggested guidelines, a majority of adults ages 20 to 74 walk less than 2 to 3 hours per week and accumulate less than 5,000 steps per day (Hedley, 2004). Pedometers and step counters are devices that track the number of steps taken per day. They are frequently used to promote daily physical activity. A meta-analysis of 26 studies evaluating pedometer use showed that PA in pedometer users increased 26.9% over baseline. Having a goal, such as 10,000 steps per day, was an important predictor of increased PA (Bravata, 2007).

Why is 10,000 steps a magic number? Adult public health guidelines for the amount of exercise required in addition to activities of daily living translate into a goal of at least 30 minutes of moderate activity per day. This is about 3,000 to 4,000 walking steps (Tudor-Locke, 2008). The idea that 10,000 steps/day is an appropriate goal for good health and weight maintenance can be traced to a promotion in Japan by pedometer companies and its adoption by walking clubs. Walking 10,000 steps is the approximate equivalent of walking 5 miles, depending on stride length. This goal may not be realistic for individuals who have been sedentary or who have chronic diseases. On the other hand, 10,000 steps/day may be too few for children or adults who are working to maintain weight loss. It seems reasonable that, instead of using a generalized 10,000 steps/day, the step goal should be based on a person's baseline plus an appropriate number of additional steps to meet health or weight management aims. For example, a healthy woman notices that she logs 4,000 steps/day on her pedometer. Her goal could be to add the equivalent of a half hour of walking to her day, or an additional 3,000 to 4,000 steps/day for a total of 7,000 to 8,000 steps. Catrine Tudor-Locke has proposed various classifications for pedometer goals in healthy adults (Tudor-Locke, 2008). These categories can be tailored to individual needs and purpose for exercising or to evaluate PA levels.

- Less than 5,000 steps/day may be defined as a "sedentary lifestyle."
- 5,000–7,499 steps/day, typical of daily activity excluding sports/exercise, could be considered "low active."

- 7,500–9,999 steps/day possibly includes some additional exercise, either purposeful or on the job, and might be considered "somewhat active."
- 10,000 steps/day indicates a classification as "active."
- Individuals who take more than 12,500 steps/day would be "highly active."

How Physical Activity Data Are Collected

The Bureau of Labor Statistics (BLS) of the United States Department of Labor annually releases the American Time Use Survey (ATUS). The BLS website shows detailed graphic and tabular presentations of current statistics on how people use their time. The data show the average amount of time per day that individuals work, do household activities, care for their children, participate in educational activities, and engage in leisure and sports activities. Data in **Figure 6.1** for 2010 show that people (age 15 years and older) who live in the United States participated in sports and

exercise activities about 19 minutes per day. In comparison to this finding, time spent watching television was 2.7 hours or roughly 8 times longer (USBLS, 2010). Trends surrounding activity levels are influenced by multiple issues including age, sex, ethnicity, socioeconomic status, education, and geographic region.

Data from the American Time Use Survey allows a closer look at the attributes of people who spend time in sports and exercise activities. An important note is that the data are self-reported from phone interviews or questionnaires and it has been shown that people are likely to overestimate their PA levels. This may be especially true for overweight individuals (Walsh, 2004).

Figure 6.2 shows that from 2003 to 2006 people living in the Pacific, New England, and Mountain regions of the United States were more likely to participate in sports or exercise activities than those in other regions. Individuals living in the Pacific region are the most likely to exercise on an average day.

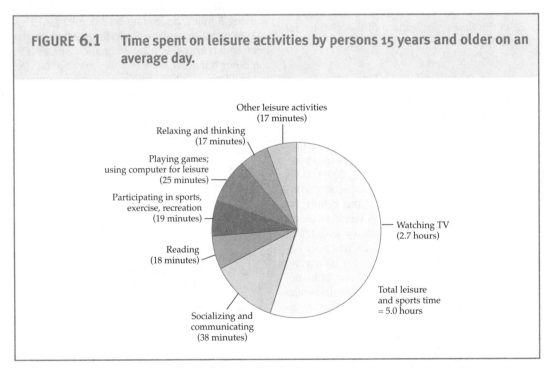

FIGURE 6.1 Time spent on leisure activities by persons 15 years and older on an average day.

Other leisure activities (17 minutes)
Relaxing and thinking (17 minutes)
Playing games; using computer for leisure (25 minutes)
Participating in sports, exercise, recreation (19 minutes)
Reading (18 minutes)
Socializing and communicating (38 minutes)
Watching TV (2.7 hours)
Total leisure and sports time = 5.0 hours

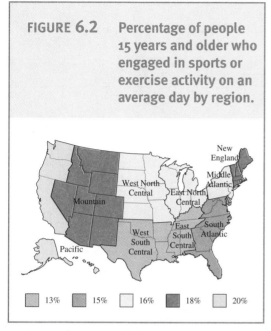

FIGURE 6.2 **Percentage of people 15 years and older who engaged in sports or exercise activity on an average day by region.**

Courtesy of: U.S. Bureau of Labor Statistics.

In general, activity decreases as people age and adequate activity is less common among women than men. The percentage of adults who do not engage in any leisure-time PA is higher among blacks (31.9%) and Latinos (34.6%) than whites (22.2%) (CDC, 2010). People living in low-income neighborhoods may have fewer resources for convenient and safe outdoor activities than those in high-income neighborhoods (Estabrooks, 2003).

As shown in **Figure 6.3**, education level is a factor in PA engagement: nearly 45% of those with a college education report some amount of regular physical activity, versus less than 20% of those who did not complete high school (USBLS, 2008).

Lack of sufficient PA is not limited to adults. Current studies show that most youth do not meet the PA guidelines for children and adolescents that recommend 60 minutes or more of moderate-to-vigorous PA per day (CDC—YRBS, 2009). Fewer children walk or bicycle to school and physical education in school has also been decreasing. Trends in school travel data published by McDonald and depicted in **Figure 6.4**, revealed that walking and biking were the most common means of getting to school in 1969 accounting for more than 40% of all trips. By 2001, active commuting to school had declined to 13%. The reduction was paralleled by a slight decline in use of school buses and public transit while the number of students driving to school increased sharply (McDonald, 2007).

An analysis of data for children and adults shows that the amount of time spent in moderate-to-vigorous PA is greatly reduced as children reach adolescence (Troiano, 2008). Data collected from

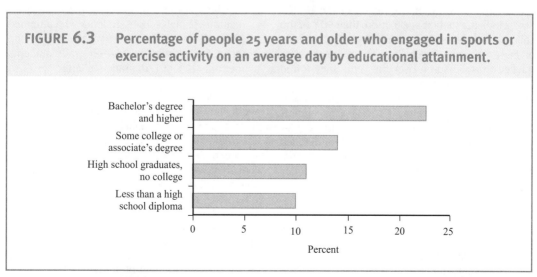

FIGURE 6.3 **Percentage of people 25 years and older who engaged in sports or exercise activity on an average day by educational attainment.**

Courtesy of: U.S. Bureau of Labor Statistics.

FIGURE 6.4 Forms of transportation to school for schoolchildren, 1965 to 2001.

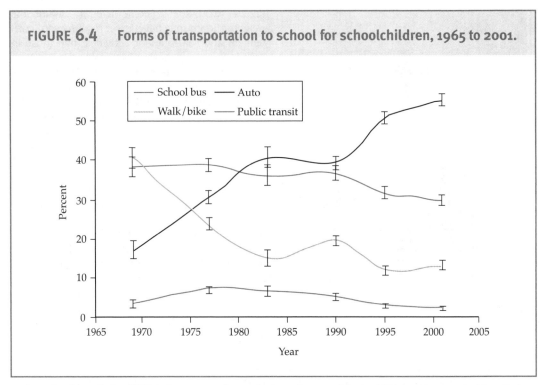

Reproduced from: McDonald NC. Active transportation to school: trends among U.S.schoolchildren, 1969–2001. *Am J Prev Med.* 2007;32(6):509–516.

more than 1,000 children from ethnically and economically diverse backgrounds in the United States indicate that, at age 9, more than 90% of the children met the recommended level of 60 minutes or more of activity each day. As the researchers tracked these children over the years they found that, by age 15, only 31% met the recommended level on weekdays, and just 17% met the recommended level on weekends (Nader, 2008). A report from a survey conducted in 2009 by the CDC—Youth Risk Behavior Surveillance System detailed participation in the more vigorous types of PA that increase heart rate or breathing rate. The agency found (CDC—YRBS, 2010):

- Eighteen percent of high school students had participated in at least 60 minutes per day of PA on each of the 7 days before the survey.
- Twenty-three percent of high school students did not participate in 60 or more minutes of PA on any day during the 7 days before the survey.

- The survey revealed that participation in PA declines as young people age. In 2009 the percentage of high school students who attended physical education classes daily during the school week was 47% of 9th grade students but only 22% of 12th grade students.

Investigators have hypothesized that electronic media may contribute to childhood obesity because sedentary media behavior displaces time that would be spent being physically active. It has also been demonstrated that children may "eat what they watch" as fat, sugar, and high-calorie food intake increases with media use (Wiecha, 2006). The CDC—Youth Risk Behavior Surveillance System (2010) assessed computer and television use in teens and found that on an average school day:

- Twenty-five percent of students played video or computer games or used a computer for something other than schoolwork for 3 or more hours.

- Thirty-three percent of students watched television 3 or more hours per day.

Recommendations for Physical Activity

The United States Department of Health and Human Services (USDHHS) *2008 Physical Activity Guidelines for Americans* (PA Guidelines) report declares that being physically active is one of the most important steps that Americans of all ages can take to improve overall health and fitness and to prevent adverse health outcomes. Evidence shows that PA can protect against diseases such as cancer, type 2 diabetes, and coronary heart disease and can increase longevity (Hu, 2004). The USDHHS issued the PA Guidelines as a complement to the USDA *Dietary Guidelines for Americans*. Taken together, they stress the importance of being physically active and eating a healthy diet to promote good health and reduce the risk of chronic diseases. The PA Guidelines focus particularly on cardiovascular and muscular fitness for the general public. The PA Guidelines do not address the activity required to improve *performance-related* fitness such as that done by competitive athletes. Current recommendations can be categorized into three groups: recommendations for good health, fitness, and to reduce the risk of chronic disease; recommendations to prevent weight gain; and recommendations to prevent weight regain after weight loss (USDHHS, 2008).

Physical Activity for Good Health, Fitness, and Prevention of Obesity

The overall message is that regular and consistent PA can produce long-term health benefits. **Table 6.2** shows adult recommendations for combining **aerobic** and **resistance** or strengthening activities. The PA Guidelines and the American College of Sports Medicine (ACSM) recommendations for PA are in weekly doses: at least the equivalent of 150 minutes per week of moderate-intensity PA for substantial health benefits, and 300 minutes per week of moderate-intensity PA for more extensive health benefits (USDHHS, 2008).

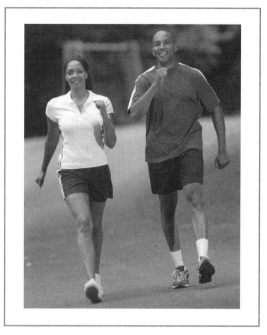

Source: © Comstock Images/Alamy Images.

The PA Guidelines also make allowances for the intensity of exercise. One and one-quarter hour of vigorous PA is approximately equal to 2.5 hours of moderate-intensity exercise. Examples of moderate-intensity aerobic activities are vigorous walking, water aerobics, ballroom dancing, and general gardening. Vigorous-intensity aerobic activities include jogging or running, swimming laps, jumping rope, and hiking uphill or with a heavy backpack. The PA Guidelines suggest that aerobic activity should be performed in episodes of at least 10 minutes. Shorter episodes of activity may be appropriate for people who have been inactive and for any adult whose ability to be active is limited. Adults should also incorporate muscle-strengthening activities such as weight training, push-ups, sit-ups, carrying heavy loads, or heavy gardening at least 2 days per week. Increasing baseline activity, or normal **lifestyle activities**, is suggested as the primary way to accumulate 150 minutes a week (CDC, 2008).

Weight maintenance is defined as weight change of less than 5%. There is considerable individual variability in response to PA and many people may need more than the equivalent of 150 minutes per

TABLE 6.2 How much physical activity do adults need?

According to the 2008 Physical Activity Guidelines for Americans, adults need to do two types of physical activity each week to improve health: aerobic and muscle-strengthening.

Adults need at least:

 2 hours and 30 minutes (150 minutes) of *moderate-intensity aerobic activity* (i.e., brisk walking) every week and *muscle-strengthening activities* on 2 or more days a week that work all major muscle groups (legs, hips, back, abdomen, chest, shoulders, and arms).

OR

 1 hour and 15 minutes (75 minutes) of *vigorous-intensity aerobic activity* (i.e., jogging or running) every week and muscle strengthening activities on 2 or more days a week that work all major muscle groups (legs, hips, back, abdomen, chest, shoulders, and arms).

OR

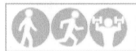 An equivalent mix of *moderate- and vigorous-intensity aerobic activity* and *muscle strengthening activities* on 2 or more days a week that will work all major muscle groups (legs, hips, abdomen, chest, shoulders, and arms).

Reproduced from: Centers for Disease Control and Prevention. How much physical activity do adults need?: CDC; 2012. http://www.cdc.gov/physicalactivity/everyone/guidelines/adults.html. *Data from*: 2008 Physical Activity Guidelines for Americans. Washington, DC: USDHHS; 2008. http://www.health.gov/paguidelines/default/aspx.

week of moderate-intensity PA to prevent weight gain and more than 300 minutes per week to initiate or maintain weight loss (USDHHS, 2008). A study of about 30,000 healthy middle-aged women found that those who do not restrict food intake need at least an hour of moderate activity a day to maintain a healthy weight (Lee, 2010). *Bottom line*: Measuring body weight is a good way to monitor whether the level of PA is sufficient to prevent weight gain. If weight increases, then more activity or fewer calories are required.

Physical Activity Recommendations for Children and Youth

Studies in children and adolescents show multiple benefits of regular physical activity. It improves strength and endurance, helps build healthy bones and muscles, helps control weight, reduces anxiety and stress, increases self-esteem, and may improve blood pressure and cholesterol levels (USDHHS, 2008). When youth have positive experiences with physical activity, it helps to build a foundation for being active throughout life. Guidelines for children

and adolescents suggest 60 minutes or more of PA daily and muscle-strengthening activities at least 3 days a week. Most of the 60 or more minutes should include either moderate- or vigorous-intensity aerobic physical activity. Examples of moderate-intensity aerobic activities include hiking, skateboarding, rollerblading, bicycle riding, and brisk walking. Vigorous-intensity aerobic activities could include jumping rope, running, and sports such as soccer, basketball, and ice or field hockey. Examples of muscle strengthening activities for younger children include gymnastics, playing on a jungle gym, and climbing a tree (USDHHS, 2008).

Physical Activity for Weight Loss

Increasing PA alone without dietary calorie reduction is not generally effective in treating obesity. Studies comparing the effectiveness of exercise and diet interventions have produced conflicting results. Only small reductions in body weight are associated with PA treatment compared to control groups who were not active. While weight loss due to PA alone has been reported with large amounts of PA, the loss is dependent on the degree of activity performed. Few studies have used a sufficient volume of PA to achieve a clinically significant degree of weight loss. The PA Guidelines for Americans report concluded that with ≥180 minutes per week of PA weight loss is typically 1 to 3% of initial body weight. With PA <150 minutes per week there is no significant reduction in body weight (USDHHS, 2008). With regard to resistance training, although it has not been shown to increase weight loss, it may increase lean mass and lower health risks. It appears that combining diet and exercise is superior to either behavior on its own (Donnelly, 2009; Jakicic, 2010). **Table 6.3** presents appropriate PA intervention strategies for weight maintenance, weight loss, and prevention of weight regain for adults.

Physical Activity to Prevent Weight Regain

Behavioral and pharmacologic treatments for obesity can lead to weight loss in most individuals in the short term. However, nearly all overweight and obese people have difficulty maintaining weight loss (Wadden, 1989). Research has shown that only about 20% of overweight individuals meet the criterion for successful weight loss, defined as losing at least 10% of initial body weight and maintaining the loss for a year or more (Wing, 2005). Even though physical exercise does not contribute greatly to weight loss, the consensus is that PA is of critical importance for weight maintenance. While there have been no well-designed, randomized, controlled trials to determine how much PA is needed to prevent weight regain after weight loss, general findings of cross-sectional and prospective studies show that weight maintenance is improved with PA of more than 250 minutes per week. Muscle-strengthening activities may help promote weight maintenance, although not to the same degree as aerobic activity (Lee, 2010). Given individual differences in response to activity, many

---

BOX 6.2   Why Do the Physical Activity Recommendations for Weight Management Seem So High?

The ineffectiveness of moderate exercise alone to reduce body fat is not surprising. Consider that 1 lb of body fat represents the equivalent of about 3,500 kcals, and to reduce body fat one must expend more energy than is consumed. An energy deficit of 500 to 1,000 kcal per day is necessary to achieve a 1- to 2-lb weight loss per week. Creating this energy deficit through PA alone is extremely difficult for most adults. Depending on body size, fitness level, and exercise intensity, an individual may burn an additional 1,000 kcal per week by exercising 30 minutes 5 days a week. In comparison, an extra 1,000 kcal could easily be consumed by miscalculating portion sizes and/or having one or two extra snacks or beverages.

- Kilocalories stored in 1 lb of body fat = 3,500 kcal
- Average kilocalories per half hour of exercise = 150 to 200 kcal
- Estimated time needed to burn a pound of body fat = 8 to 12 hours

Kilocalories in:
   1 medium sesame seed bagel = 290 kcal
   2 Tbsp of peanut butter = 180 kcal
   20-oz bottle of regular cola = 240 kcal

By entering weight, age, sex, and activity duration, online activity calorie counters can be used to calculate the number of calories an individual needs to perform various activities. Check the websites listed in the Resources section in this chapter to find these calculators.

TABLE 6.3	Physical Activity Recommendations for Weight Management
Weight maintenance:	• PA of 150–250 min/week (using an energy equivalent of 1,200–2,000 kcal/week) will prevent weight gain in most adults.
Weight loss:	• PA of less than 150 min/week will result in minimal weight loss.
	• There is generally a dose-response effect of PA on weight loss.
	• Greater weight loss and enhanced prevention of weight regain occurs with PA of 250–300 min/week (at least 2,000 kcal/week) of moderate-intensity PA.*
Weight regain prevention:	• Approximately 200–300 min/week may help minimize weight regain after weight loss.
	• No well-designed studies provide evidence concerning the amount of PA needed to prevent weight regain.
	• The consensus is that more PA is required to prevent weight regain compared with weight maintenance.
Resistance training:	• Resistance training is ineffective for weight loss with or without diet restriction, according to limited research evidence.
	• Muscle-strengthening activities may help promote weight maintenance, although not to the same degree as aerobic activity.
	• Resistance training may enhance lean mass protection and increase loss of body fat during energy restriction.
	• Resistance training may also reduce occurrence of risk factors for chronic disease, such as abnormal cholesterol levels and insulin resistance.

*Moderate-intensity activity as 3.0 to 5.9 metabolic equivalents.

Data from: Donnelly JE, Blair SN, Jakicic JM, Manore MM, Rankin JW, Smith BK. American College of Sports Medicine Position Stand. Appropriate physical activity intervention strategies for weight loss and prevention of weight regain for adults. *Med Sci Sports Exerc.* Feb 2009;41(2):459–471.

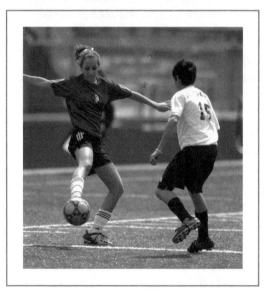

Source: © Shawn Pecor/ShutterStock, Inc.

people who are trying to keep a significant amount of weight off once it has been lost may need to do more than 300 minutes (5 hours) a week of moderate-intensity activity to meet weight management goals (USDHHS, 2008). Further, evidence indicates that individuals who are successful at long-term weight maintenance, such as those in the National Weight Control Registry (NWCR), report that they limit caloric intake in addition to maintaining physical activity.

Physical Activity and the National Weight Control Registry Participants

The NWCR tracks thousands of individuals who have successfully maintained weight loss. The participants report using a variety of methods to lose weight, but for more than 90% some kind of PA is a key aspect of their long-term weight-loss maintenance. Individuals in the NWCR who have

---

BOX 6.3 National Weight Control Registry (NWCR)

The NWCR was established in 1993 to investigate characteristics and behaviors of individuals who have been successful at long-term weight-loss maintenance. With about 5,000 participants, the NWCR is the largest longitudinal prospective study of those who have lost significant amounts of weight and kept it off for long periods of time. Detailed questionnaires and annual follow-up surveys are used to examine the behavioral and psychological characteristics of weight maintainers, as well as the strategies they use to maintain their weight losses. To qualify for NWCR entry, individuals must have lost a minimum of 13.6 kg (30 lb) and have maintained that amount of weight loss for at least 1 year. The Resources section in this chapter lists websites with more information about how to register and to learn more about the eating and exercise habits of successful weight losers and the behavioral strategies they use to maintain their weight.

---

maintained weight loss have an average weekly energy expenditure equivalent to moderate-speed walking of 28 miles or more than 2,800 kcal. However, there is substantial variability in the amount of PA reported as 25% reported that they performed activities equal to less than 1,000 kcal/week and 35% reported energy expenditure greater than 3,000 kcal/week. While the NWCR participants are generally a physically active group, the variability of their activity levels makes it difficult to set specific recommendations for the optimum amount of PA necessary for weight-loss maintenance (Catenacci, 2008).

Benefits, Risks, and Costs of Physical Activity

It is easier to achieve a calorie deficit with diet rather than by exercise, but exercise is not futile or ineffective in obesity management. Strong evidence shows that physically active adults who are overweight or obese experience health benefits that are associated with those observed in people with optimal body weight. These benefits include lower rates of all-cause mortality, coronary heart disease, hypertension, stroke, type 2 diabetes, colon cancer, and breast cancer. In the Nurses' Health Study, which followed 116,564 women for 24 years, increased body fat and low PA were both strong, independent predictors of death. Compared

with lean active women, the percentage increase in death from all causes was 155% for lean inactive women; 191% for obese active women; and 245% for obese inactive women (Hu, 2004). **Table 6.4** provides a summary of the health benefits strongly associated with regular physical activity. Many of these benefits appear to be independent of body weight.

Owing to the health benefits of PA that are independent of body weight classification, the PA Guidelines declare that "adults of all sizes and shapes gain health and fitness benefits by being habitually physically active" (USDHHS—report, 2008). Given the advantages of activity for any size person, health professionals promote the health benefits of exercise independent of body weight and shift the focus from changes in body weight to changes in overall physical and psychological well-being (King, 2009).

Metabolic Health

Excess fat deposits around the abdomen or visceral adipose tissue (VAT) has been linked to abnormal blood concentrations of glucose, insulin, and lipids. Increased VAT is also associated with development of atherosclerosis, type 2 diabetes, cardiovascular disease, and stroke (Tresierras, 2009). There is some evidence that regular PA can alter body composition and fat distribution, particularly by reducing VAT as measured by a decrease in waist

TABLE 6.4   Health Benefits Strongly Associated with Regular Physical Activity

Children and Adolescents

Improved cardiorespiratory and muscular fitness

Improved bone health

Improved cardiovascular and metabolic health biomarkers

Favorable body composition

Adults and Older Adults

Lower risk of early death

Lower risk of coronary heart disease

Lower risk of stroke

Lower risk of high blood pressure

Lower risk of adverse blood lipid profile

Lower risk of type 2 diabetes

Lower risk of metabolic syndrome

Lower risk of colon cancer

Lower risk of breast cancer

Prevention of weight gain

Weight loss, particularly when combined with reduced calorie intake

Improved cardiorespiratory and muscular fitness

Prevention of falls

Reduced depression

Better cognitive function (for older adults)

Note: The Advisory Committee rated the evidence from studies of health benefits of physical activity as strong, moderate, or weak. This table includes those benefits that fall into the "Strong evidence" category.

Reproduced from: Physical Activity Guidelines Advisory Committee Report, 2008. Courtesy of the U.S. Department of Health and Human Services.

circumference (WC) measurement in both men and women. A number of studies suggest that PA may counterbalance the hazardous health effects of increased adiposity, and reduced visceral fat mass may be the key factor associated with individuals who are obese, but metabolically healthy (Lee, 2009). These beneficial changes have been observed with and without calorie-restriction diets (Tresierras, 2009). In addition, VAT and WC can be significantly reduced in response to exercise even without weight reduction (van der Heijden, 2010). Given these data that show that higher levels of fitness may reduce morbidity and mortality in obese patients, increasing PA would be an effective lifestyle intervention, particularly for people with obesity who are unable to achieve or maintain weight loss. These reports of metabolic benefits without a reduction in calorie intake or body weight bring up the question of whether weight loss is the best outcome for determining the success of treatment strategies to reduce obesity and related comorbidities. It may be that the question about which is more important, inactivity or obesity, is beside the point. The imperative for both conditions is to increase PA (Lee, 2009).

Risks

The 2008 PA Guidelines Committee Report reviewed studies concerning the risk of **musculoskeletal** injury and other adverse events related to PA and assessed whether the benefits of regular PA outweigh the risks. Physical activity–related adverse events are defined as undesired health events that occur because a person is physically active. They may be mild or severe and include conditions such as musculoskeletal injuries or cardiac events. The most common risk of PA in adults is musculoskeletal injury. Risk of injury increases with participation in contact or collision sports, such as soccer or football, while noncontact physical activity, such as walking for exercise, gardening or yard work, dancing, swimming, and golf, are activities with the lowest injury rates. However, inactive individuals are more likely to be injured than people who exercise regularly when performing the same activity (USDHHS, 2008). Cardiac events, such as a heart attack or sudden death during physical activity, are rare though the risk of such events does increase when a person suddenly becomes much more active than usual. The greatest risk occurs when an inactive adult engages in a vigorous-intensity activity such as shoveling snow. Research findings show that people who are consistently physically active have the lowest risk of cardiac events during activity or at rest (Thompson, 2003).

Vigorous PA may increase the risk of cardiac abnormalities among individuals with diagnosed heart disease. Hence, the often-stated caution is to check with a physician before beginning a new exercise program. It is interesting that the PA Guidelines Committee Report states that men and women who do not have symptoms of heart disease may prudently and reasonably increase their daily physical activities without the need to consult a healthcare provider before doing so. The incidence of activity-related cardiovascular or musculoskeletal adverse events has not been shown to be reduced by a medical consultation. The available scientific literature suggests that adding a comfortable amount of light- to moderate-intensity activity, such as walking two to three times per week, has a low risk of musculoskeletal injury and no known risk of sudden severe cardiac events (USDHHS—report, 2008).

Even though occurrence, or fear, of adverse events may prevent participation in regular physical activity, the bottom line is that the health benefits of PA outweigh the risks. Physically active people have lower all-cause mortality rates, lower risk of chronic disease, and lower medical expenditures. Choosing low-risk activities and sensible behavior while doing any activity can minimize the frequency and severity of adverse events and maximize the benefits of regular physical activity.

Costs

The costs of being physically active include time, effort, and sometimes money. Opportunity costs are the value of an alternate activity that is replaced to spend time and physical exertion exercising. There may be costs to purchase fitness equipment or to join a gym or health club. Health economists have noted that in earlier agricultural and industrial times, energy expenditure was part of one's daily work. Today physical labor is not always built in to everyday life and people must allot time and money resources for exercise (Variyam, 2005).

Summary

Maintaining energy balance is the key factor that determines whether a person can prevent weight loss or gain. Energy consumed as food and energy expended in PA both contribute to energy balance. Low levels of PA are associated with increased risk of overweight and obesity. Whether a person is active or not is influenced by such demographic issues as age, sex, ethnicity, and even where an individual lives. Current PA trends in the United States indicate that more than half of the adult population does not meet PA requirement for good health. While a large percentage of children do get adequate PA, the time spent in PA declines sharply as they grow to adolescence and young adulthood.

The 2008 PA Guidelines stress the importance of regular PA to promote good health, lowered risk of chronic conditions such as cardiovascular disease and type 2 diabetes, and for weight management. It is reasonable that the amount of PA required to maintain weight is less than that needed to either lose weight or to keep weight off after weight reduction. However, it is surprising that moderate exercise alone is not sufficient to produce significant weight loss. Both calorie restriction and increased PA must be combined to create a negative energy balance that will cause weight loss. PA is very effective at helping to prevent weight regain. Individuals in the NWCR report that PA is an essential aspect of long-term weight management. PA has many health advantages that occur even in the absence of weight loss or calorie restriction. Consistent PA on its own is linked to lower blood pressure and cholesterol, less anxiety and depression, and a lower risk of early death and disease. Experts concur that the exercise component of a lifestyle intervention should focus primarily on improving metabolic fitness and decreasing disease risk independent of weight loss.

Critical Thinking Questions

Question: What is the nature of the association of PA with energy balance? Focus on differences among:
- Weight maintenance (having less than 3% change in weight).
- Weight loss (achieving at least 5% loss of weight).
- Weight maintenance following weight loss.

Question: Walking 10,000 steps is the approximate equivalent of walking 5 miles. Discuss the various factors that explain why this is just an approximation.

Question: If weight loss is not the only benefit of exercise, nor is it the most useful and appropriate marker of health, can a person be both fit and fat?

Question: The PA Guidelines suggest that the most effective way to accumulate at least 150 minutes PA each week is to increase baseline activities or normal lifestyle activities. Brainstorm or describe effective interventions that could help develop a contemporary culture where PA is the social norm.

Activity: Use the About.com Walking website (http://walking.about.com/library/cal/uccalc1.htm) to assess calories burned during exercise.

With the Walking Calories Calculator:
a. Figure out the calories burned for a 150-lb woman who walks for 2 miles at 3 miles per hour (mph).
b. Figure out the calories she burns when she walks for 2 miles at 4 mph.
c. What would the calories be if she walked for 3 miles at 3 mph?
d. What would the calories be if she walked for 3 miles at 4 mph?
e. Considering the time it takes and the calories burned, what do you think is the most effective or most realistic walking plan for this woman?

Resources

The National Weight Control Registry

http://www.nwcr.ws/

The NWCR was developed to identify and investigate the characteristics of individuals who have succeeded at long-term weight loss

Websites with Activity Calculators to Check Calories Burned

http://www.caloriescount.com

http://www.fitday.com

http://www.primusweb.com/fitnesspartner/calculat.htm

By selecting an activity and entering your weight, these calculators tell the energy required for various physical activities.

Shape Up America!

http://www.shapeup.org/index.html

This is an organization that educates the public on the importance of a healthy body weight through PA and healthy eating. Check the website for nutrition and PA tips for adults and children and to find out more about the 10,000 steps program.

CDC KidsWalk-to-School.

http://www.cdc.gov/nccdphp/dnpa/kidswalk/then_and_now.htm

To support the national goal of better health through physical activity, CDC's Nutrition and PA Program has developed KidsWalk-to-School, a community-based program that aims to increase opportunities for daily PA by encouraging children to walk to and from school in groups accompanied by adults.

2008 Physical Activity Guidelines for Americans.

http://www.health.gov/paguidelines/

The United States Department of Health and Human Services *Physical Activity Guidelines* describe the types and amounts of PA that offer substantial health benefits to Americans.

CDC Healthy Youth Health Topics

http://www.cdc.gov/HealthyYouth

The National Youth Risk Behavior Survey (YRBS) monitors priority health risk behaviors that contribute to the leading causes of death, disability, and social problems among youth and adults in the United States. Check the Trends in the Prevalence of Physical Activity on this site.

American Time Use Survey.

http://www.bls.gov/tus/

The American Time Use Survey (ATUS) provides statistics and graphical data on the amount of time people in the United States spend on various activities that provide a snapshot of how Americans spend their days.

References

Bravata DM, Smith-Spangler C, Sundaram V, Gienger AL, Lin N, Lewis R, Stave CD, Olkin I, Sirard JR. Using pedometers to increase physical activity and improve health: a systematic review. *JAMA*. 2007;298: 2296–2304.

Catenacci VA, Ogden LG, Stuht J, et al. Physical activity patterns in the National Weight Control Registry. *Obesity (Silver Spring)*. Jan 2008;16(1):153–161.

CDC. Centers for Disease Control and Prevention. 2008 U.S. Physical Activity Statistics: Summary of Physical Activity. 2008; http://apps.nccd.cdc.gov/PASurveillance/StateSumV.asp Accessed March 22, 2010.

CDC. Centers for Disease Control and Prevention. 2009 Physical Activity for a Healthy Weight. http://www.cdc.gov/healthyweight/physical_activity/index.html. Accessed July 2010.

CDC. Centers for Disease Control and Prevention. Youth Risk Behavior Surveillance—United States, 2009. *Morbidity and Mortality Weekly Report*. 2010; 59(SS-5); http://www.cdc.gov/mmwr/pdf/ss/ss5905.pdf. Accessed September, 2010.

Donnelly JE, Blair SN, Jakicic JM, et al. American College of Sports Medicine. American College of Sports Medicine Position Stand. Appropriate physical activity intervention strategies for weight loss and prevention of weight regain for adults. *Med Sci Sports Exerc*. 2009;41:459–471.

Elfhag K, Rossner S. Who succeeds in maintaining weight loss? A conceptual review of factors associated with weight loss maintenance and weight regain. *Obes Rev*. Feb 2005;6(1):67–85.

Estabrooks PA, Lee RE, Gyurcsik NC. Resources for physical activity participation: does availability and accessibility differ by neighborhood socioeconomic status? *Ann Behav Med.* Spring 2003;25(2):100–104.

Haapanen N, Miilunpalo S, Pasanen M, Oja P, Vuori I. Association between leisure time physical activity and 10-year body mass change among working-aged men and women. *Int J Obes Relat Metab Disord.* Apr 1997;21(4):288-296.

Hedley AA, Ogden CL, Johnson CL, Carroll MD, Curtin LR, Flegal KM. Prevalence of overweight and obesity among US children, adolescents, and adults, 1999–2002. *JAMA.* Jun 16 2004;291(23):2847-2850.

Hu FB, Willett WC, Li T, et al. Adiposity as compared with physical activity in predicting mortality among women. *N Engl J Med.* 2004;351:2694-2703.

Jakicic JM, Otto AD, Lang W, et al. The effect of physical activity on 18-month weight change in overweight adults. Obesity (Silver Spring). Jan 2011;19(1):100–109.

King NA, Hopkins M, Caudwell P, Stubbs RJ, Blundell JE. Beneficial effects of exercise: shifting the focus from body weight to other markers of health. *Br J Sports Med.* Dec 2009;43(12):924-927.

Lee IM, Djoussé L, Sesso HD, et al. Physical activity and weight gain prevention. *JAMA.* 2010;303(12): 1173-1179.

Lee DC, Sui X, Blair SN. Does physical activity ameliorate the health hazards of obesity? *Br J Sports Med.* 2009;43(1):9-51.

McDonald NC. Active transportation to school: trends among U.S. schoolchildren, 1969–2001. *Am J Prev Med.* 2007;32(6):509-516.

Nader PR, Bradley RH, Houts RM, McRitchie SL, O'Brien M. Moderate-to-vigorous physical activity from ages 9 to 15 years. *JAMA.* Jul 16 2008;300(3):295-305.

Shape Up America. Getting started on the 10,000 Steps Program. 2010; http://www.shapeup.org/index .html. Accessed August 2010.

Thompson PD, Buchner D, Piña IL, Balady GJ, Williams MA, Marcus BH, et al. Exercise and physical activity in the prevention and treatment of atherosclerotic cardiovascular disease: a statement from the Council on Clinical Cardiology (Subcommittee on Exercise, Rehabilitation, and Prevention) and the Council on Nutrition, Physical Activity, and Metabolism (Subcommittee on Physical Activity). *Circulation.* 2003;107:3109-3116.

Tresierras, MA, Balady GJ. Resistance training in the treatment of diabetes and obesity: mechanisms and

outcomes. *J Cardiopulm Rehabil Prev.* 2009;29(2): 67-75.

Troiano R, Berrigan D, Dodd K, et al. Physical activity in the United States measured by accelerometer. *Med Sci Sports Exer.* 2008;40(1):181-188.

Tudor-Locke C, Hatano Y, Pangrazi RP, Kang M. Revisiting "how many steps are enough?" *Med Sci Sports Exerc.* Jul 2008;40(7 Suppl):S537-543.

USBLS. American Time Use Survey—2009 Results. 2010; http://www.bls.gov/news.release/pdf/atus.pdf. Accessed July 2011.

USBLS. American Time Use. Sports and Exercise. 2008; http://www.bls.gov/tus/. Accessed August 2010.

USDHHS—report. U.S. Department of Health and Human Services. Physical Activity Guidelines Advisory Committee Report. 2008; http://www.health.gov/ paguidelines/. Accessed March 31, 2010.

USDHHS. U.S. Department of Health and Human Services. *2008 Physical Activity Guidelines for Americans.*2; http://www.health.gov/paguidelines/. Accessed August 2009.

van der Heijden GJ, Wang ZJ, Chu ZD, et al. A 12-week aerobic exercise program reduces hepatic fat accumulation and insulin resistance in obese, Hispanic adolescents. *Obesity (Silver Spring).* Feb 2010;18(2):384-390.

Variyam JN. The Price is Right: Economics and the Rise in Obesity. AmberWaves 2005(February, 2005). http://www.ers.usda.gov/AmberWaves/February05/Features/ThePriceIsRight.htm.

Wadden TA, Sternberg JA, Letizia KA, Stunkard AJ, Foster GD. Treatment of obesity by very low calorie diet, behavior therapy, and their combination: a five-year perspective. *Int J Obes.* 1989;13 Suppl 2: 39-46.

Walsh MC, Hunter GR, Sirikul B, et al. Comparison of self-reported with objectively assessed energy expenditure in black and white women before and after weight loss. *Am J Clin Nutr.* 2004;79:1013-1019.

Wiecha JL, Peterson KE, Ludwig DS, Kim J, Sobol A, Gortmaker SL. When children eat what they watch: impact of television viewing on dietary intake in youth. *Arch Pediatr Adolesc Med.* Apr 2006;160(4):436-442.

Wing RR, Hill JO. Successful weight loss maintenance. *Annu Rev Nutr.* 2001;21:323-341.

Wing, RR, Phelan S. Long-term weight loss maintenance. *Am J Clin Nutr.* 2005;82(1 Suppl): 222S-225S.

CHAPTER 7

PHARMACOLOGIC AGENTS IN OBESITY MANAGEMENT

READER OBJECTIVES

- Describe the indication and incidence of prescription medications for weight loss
- Recognize the benefits and drawbacks associated with prescription medication regulation
- Explain the two types of physiologic action of currently approved drugs for weight management
- Discuss the safety and efficacy of currently available obesity medication and apply the concept of off-label use
- Describe realistic goals of pharmacotherapy for weight management
- Compare and contrast the regulation, safety, and efficacy of prescription medications with over-the-counter drugs and supplements marketed for weight loss

CHAPTER OUTLINE

Medications for Weight Loss

The problem of weight control is complex, and it requires a combination of lifestyle, behavioral, and dietary changes to manage effectively. While the appropriate number of calories and regular exercise are essential to successful weight management, for some, antiobesity drugs may be a helpful addition to enhance weight loss. Because most obese individuals are not successful in their attempts to lose weight and keep it off (Jeffery, 2000), the case for safe and effective **pharmacotherapy** is evident. However, the current drugs available for long-term weight management are limited in number and efficacy, and pharmacotherapy for obesity has seen many challenges and setbacks. While many drugs have been approved for the treatment of obesity, most have also been withdrawn due to serious side effects.

In the early 1900s, people seeking a treatment for obesity were given doses of such things as vinegar and soap. This type of ingredient produced almost instant, though short-lived, weight reduction because it acted as a laxative that caused diarrhea and a purgative that produced vomiting. Other highly advertised weight-loss drugs were concoctions of animal-derived thyroid, arsenic, or strychnine. Each could cause temporary weight loss but they were obviously unsafe over the long term. For decades thyroid hormone was medically prescribed for obesity with the hope that an increase in metabolic rate would help with weight loss. However, thyroid as an active ingredient increased risk of hypertension, cardiac arrest, and stroke. Long-term use could result in loss of normal thyroid function, osteoporosis, chest pain, and sudden death. The American Medical Association was eventually successful in getting the thyroid extract removed from these diet products.

Another interesting diet prescription in the 1930s was Dinitrophenol, a benzene-derived ingredient in World War I explosives. Dinitrophenol did in fact increase metabolism and produce weight loss, but the drug had to be abandoned because of severe side effects including cataracts and nerve damage. Dextroamphetamine, developed as a treatment for narcolepsy, was marketed as a weight-loss drug in 1937 when it was discovered that it could reduce appetite as well as keep people awake. For decades, amphetamines were a popular weight-loss therapy and for good reason—they worked. Amphetamines were not without risks. The drug is associated with accelerated heart rate, increased blood pressure, hallucinations, psychiatric disorders, addiction, and withdrawal problems. These side effects brought about the end of the amphetamine era. In the 1970s government agencies around the world adopted tighter restrictions on these types of drugs with the potential for abuse. Amphetamines are no longer widely prescribed or available over the counter, but they are still used with tight regulations in many countries today. In the 1990s, as a response to increased rates of obesity, there was another great interest in the use of **anorectics**. It was at that time that the "Fen-Phen" drug combination became instantly (although briefly) popular (Stafford, 2003).

Incidence: How Many People Use Weight-Loss Medications?

According to the American Society of Bariatric Physicians (ASBP) 2008 survey of bariatric specialists, 97% reported that they prescribed pharmacotherapy for their patients with weight management goals (Steelman, 2010). That is not the case with medical practitioners in general. Negative publicity received by weight-loss medications that have been withdrawn from the market as a result of serious side effects has greatly discouraged physicians from prescribing them. As a result, the percentage of Americans who use antiobesity drugs has been declining. From a peak of nearly 10 million prescriptions for the medications in 1997, their use diminished to about 3 million in 2002 following the removal of the popular drug Fenfluramine from the market (Stafford, 2003). A 2009 article in the journal *Obesity* reported that among the 4.2 million persons enrolled in Blue Cross and Blue Shield plans, the number of persons who took an antiobesity medication decreased from 1% in 2002 to 0.7% in 2005 (Bolen, 2010).

How Are Prescription Weight-Loss Medications Regulated?

In 1938 the United States Congress passed the Federal Food, Drug, and Cosmetic Act giving authority to the Food and Drug Administration (FDA) to oversee the safety of food, drugs, and cosmetics before they can be put on the market. In the case of prescription weight-loss medications the FDA's regulatory authority includes oversight of development and testing, approval, monitoring safety once the drug is released, and, if necessary, product recalls. It was not until 1996 that the FDA issued clear guidelines for the development of obesity drugs with the release of the publication, "Guidance for the Clinical Evaluation of Weight-Control Drugs." An updated version was published in 2007 giving "recommendations for the design and conduct of clinical studies aimed at demonstrating the effectiveness and safety of weight-loss medications" (FDA, 2007). The guide gives the following recommendations:

- Weight control by new drugs must be demonstrated over 1 year to classify a product as being effective.
- Weight loss induced by the drug must be ≥5% compared with a placebo.
- The percentage of drug-treated subjects losing ≥5% of baseline body weight must be ≥35% and double the percentage from the placebo-treated subjects.
- At least 3,000 subjects must be assigned to the experimental drug with no fewer than 1,500 subjects assigned to placebo for a 1-year period to satisfy safety concerns.

In addition, the FDA mandated BMI restrictions in clinical trials for antiobesity drugs (Steelman, 2010). Pharmacotherapy is recommended as a weight-loss treatment option for persons with either a BMI of 30 or more who have no obesity-related conditions, or a BMI of 27 or more with two or more obesity-related conditions such as type 2 diabetes, sleep apnea, or hypertension. In all cases, it is recommended that risk/benefit of pharmacotherapy be assessed (NHLBI, 1998; FDA, 2007).

While these regulatory guidelines promote drug safety and efficacy, they do demand a huge investment of time and resources from biopharmaceutical companies that may have contributed to the lack of new antiobesity drugs currently available to physicians and their patients. In addition, in the last few years many drugs that have been effective weight-loss medications have had to be withdrawn from the market due to adverse side effects. Fen-Phen, which was marketed as a combination of two drugs Fenfluramine and Phentermine, was removed from the market in September 1997, after it was reported that it could cause valvular heart disease and pulmonary hypertension (Connolly, 1997). Some of the newer drugs in development for weight loss work by modifying brain chemistry. This approach can have unintended consequences, as was the case of rimonabant. The medication changes brain chemistry to make eating less pleasurable and reduce food cravings. The weight-loss data was impressive but, for some individuals, taking away eating pleasure lead to depression. Rimonabant was never approved in the United States but was available for a time in Europe before being withdrawn in 2008 after a series of suicides in people who took the drug (Leite, 2009).

More recently, in October 2010, Sibutramine, a serotonin-norepinephrine reuptake inhibitor, was withdrawn from the market because of its association with increased cardiovascular events and strokes (James, 2010). Because of lack of long-term data on safety and effectiveness, most of the drugs approved for obesity have been approved for short-term use only. A list of FDA approved obesity drugs can be viewed in **Table 7.1**.

Pharmacologic Mechanisms of Prescription Weight-Loss Medications

Products That Work Systemically as Appetite Suppressants

Phentermine, Diethylpropion, Phendimetrazine, and Benzphetamine are amphetamine-derived

---

BOX 7.1 Alternate Opinion of the American Society of Bariatric Physicians on Weight-Loss Medications

---

The ASBP obesity medication recommendations vary from the FDA short-term use only guidelines. The professional group of bariatric physicians proposes that anorectic agents may be part of a lifelong weight-maintenance program as long as they continue to bring about a beneficial clinical response, which may be defined as:

1. Loss of weight (an average of at least 1.4 kg, or about 3 lb, per month of therapy has been suggested).
2. Loss of 10% of maximum (nonpregnant) weight in a healthy patient qualifying for initiation criteria.
3. Loss of 5% of maximum (nonpregnant) weight in patients who are at increased risk because of associated comorbidities.

Source: ASBP. American Society of Bariatric Physicians. Overweight and Obesity Evaluation and Management. 2009; http://www.asbp.org/resources. Accessed April 10, 2011.

TABLE 7.1 FDA Approved Obesity Drugs

Drug	Trade name examples	Year approved	Year withdrawn from market
Short-term use: Drugs that are sympathomimetic amines and similar to amphetamines			
Phentermine	Ionamin, Fastin, Adipex-P	1959	2000 in EU
Diethylpropion	Tenuate	1959	
Phendimetrazine	Bontril, Plegine	1959	
Benzphetamine	Didrex	1960	
Mazindol	Sanorex	1973	
Short-term use: Drugs that increase serotonin levels			
Fenfluramine	Pondimin	1973	1997
Long-term use: Drugs that increase serotonin levels			
Dexfenfluramine	Redux	1996	1997
Sibutramine	Meridia	1997	2010
Long-term use: Drugs that inhibit intestinal lipases			
Orlistat	alli, Xenical	1999	

medications that can promote weight loss by decreasing appetite and/or increasing satiety. Although the mechanism of action of these sympathetic nervous-system-stimulating, or **sympathomimetic**, drugs in the treatment of obesity is not fully known, these medications are thought to suppress appetite through inhibition of **neurotransmitter** recycling. This leads to increased extracellular concentrations of norepinephrine and epinephrine **monoamines** that act as hormones and neurotransmitters. These sympathomimetic amines, which are similar to amphetamines, stimulate the central nervous system, which increases heart rate and blood pressure and activates the fight-or-flight response. In addition, they cause a decrease in appetite. Because neurotransmitters regulate a wide variety of functions, these drugs may carry risks of addiction, hypertension, and cardiovascular disturbances (Sargent, 2009). Phentermine and Diethylpropion are most commonly prescribed due to their reduced potential for addiction (Robinson, 2009). They are approved for short-term use (12 weeks) for weight loss. That means they actually have limited use for long-term obesity management.

Products That Inhibit Absorption of Fat from the Gastrointestinal Tract

The lipase inhibitor Orlistat is a class of weight-loss drugs that works by binding to the active sites of gastric and pancreatic lipases in the gastrointestinal tract. Because enzyme activity is blocked, a significant proportion of dietary fat is unable to be absorbed and it passes through the GI tract unchanged. See **Figure 7.1** for a visualization of how a lipase inhibitor functions. At the recommended therapeutic dose, Orlistat can inhibit absorption of up to 30% of dietary fat. Theoretically, the reduction in fat digestion may reduce total energy intake to produce weight loss.

Availability of Prescription Medications for Weight Loss/ Management

Sympathomimetic drugs and lipase inhibitors are the only two types of obesity medications that are currently approved by the FDA. The sole FDA-approved drug for long-term use is Orlistat,

which is available in both prescription and OTC forms.

Appetite Suppressants

Most available weight-loss medications are amphetamine-derivative sympathomimetic appetite suppressants. Phentermine, which has been available since the late 1950s, is the most commonly prescribed weight-loss medication in the United States. It is approved for short-term use and it has been evaluated as both monotherapy and as combination therapy. However, data from a long-term randomized clinical trial of Phentermine monotherapy are not available (Hendricks, 2009). A 1-year randomized double-blind placebo-controlled study showed that a similar drug, Diethylpropion, was safe and effective. In addition to a calorie-controlled diet, 69 obese healthy adults were randomized to Diethylpropion or placebo for 6 months. For the following 6 months all participants received the drug. During the first 6 months, the treatment group lost nearly 10% of initial body weight versus about 3% in the placebo group. When all participants were taking the drug, at 12 months both groups had lost 7 to 10% of initial body weight, and the difference between groups was not significant. In addition, there was no difference between the two groups with respect to cardiovascular and psychiatric side effects (Cercato, 2009).

Phentermine and Diethylpropion are approved for short-term treatment, which usually is interpreted as up to 12 weeks. However, these medications have been shown to reduce weight significantly when used intermittently (Munro, 1968). This means that they could possibly be used as chronic medications while complying with the short-term limitations as long as they are used in alternating months. The main side effects of these drugs are insomnia, dry mouth, and constipation. Experts caution that individuals with heart disease, high blood pressure, an overactive thyroid gland, or glaucoma should not use these drugs (WIN, 2010). However, data from a recent study suggest that hypertension associated with Phentermine pharmacotherapy is rare rather than common (Hendricks, 2011).

Two other types of appetite suppressant drugs that were effective for weight management are no longer available. The Fenfluramine and Dexfenfluramine groups are pharmacologically similar

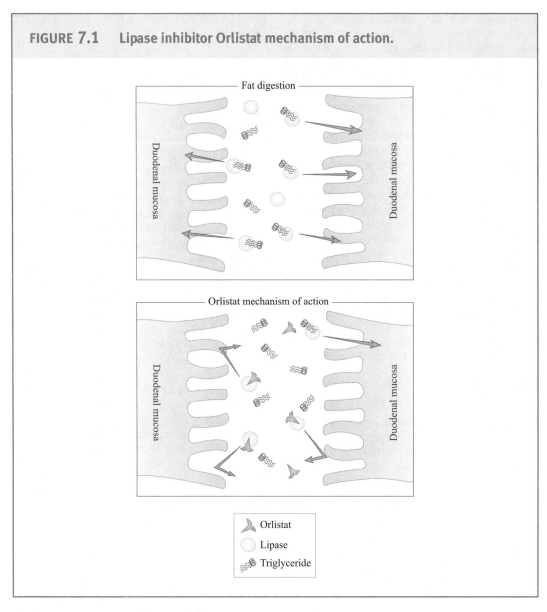

FIGURE 7.1   Lipase inhibitor Orlistat mechanism of action.

to antidepressants and worked by promoting the release of **serotonin** and inhibiting its reuptake. By altering serotonin levels, the Fenfluramines allowed users to experience positive feelings and a reduced appetite. Fenfluramine and Dexfenfluramine were withdrawn from the market in 1997 by recommendation of the FDA. These drugs used alone and in combination with Phentermine (Fen-Phen) were linked to the development of valvular heart disease and primary pulmonary hypertension, a rare but potentially fatal disorder that affects the blood vessels in the lungs (WIN, 2010). Sibutramine (Meridia), a popular drug in the noradrenergic/serotonergic category, was voluntarily withdrawn from United States and Canadian markets in October 2010. Data from a postmarketing study, the Sibutramine

Cardiovascular Outcomes (SCOUT) Trial, indicated that individuals with cardiovascular disease had an increased risk of heart attack and stroke with this drug (James, 2010).

Lipase Inhibitors

Orlistat (Xenical) is the only weight-loss medication allowed for long-term use in obesity treatment. Clinical trials have demonstrated that Orlistat can produce weight loss that can be sustained for up to 2 years (Davidson, 1999). Meta-analysis of clinical trials indicates that patients treated with Orlistat displayed a 2.89 kg (6 lb) or a 3% greater reduction in weight than placebo-treated patients after a 1-year follow-up (Rucker, 2007). In 2004, the FDA approved Orlistat use for the treatment of obesity among adolescents, thereby making it the first approved weight-loss treatment for children and adolescents in the United States. In 2007, Orlistat was approved for OTC sale for adults age 18 years and older. The version of Orlistat sold under the brand name alli may be purchased without a prescription. Both drugs contain different strengths of Orlistat as Xenical contains 120 mg, whereas alli contains 60 mg. Either type of Orlistat is meant to be taken with a reduced-calorie, low-fat diet. Because Orlistat reduces the absorption of lipid-soluble vitamins (A, D, E, and K), patients are advised to take a multivitamin at least 2 hours before or after taking Orlistat.

With Orlistat, up to 30% of ingested fat is not absorbed. This is the reason for the most common adverse events that may include oily spotting, liquid stools, fecal urgency or incontinence, flatulence, and abdominal cramping. These side effects are generally mild and temporary, but may be worsened by eating high-fat foods. It may be that the benefit of the drug is enhanced in patients who learn to switch to a low-fat diet to avoid such side effects. A few cases of severe liver injury have been reported in patients using either Xenical or alli. According to the FDA Postmarket Drug Safety Information for Patients and Providers, out of an estimated 40 million people worldwide who have used Xenical or alli, one case of liver injury with alli in the United States and 12 foreign cases with Xenical were reported. A causal relationship between this drug and liver disorders has not been established; however, the FDA has approved revised labeling for both drugs and recommends that clinicians consider the risks and benefits of pharmacotherapy with these drugs before prescribing or suggesting therapy with either formulation. Information about Orlistat and liver injury is available on the FDA drug safety website listed in the Resources section in this chapter.

The combination of only modest weight loss and undesirable side effects leads to high attrition rates in users. Less than 1% of patients still take the drug after 1 year and only 2% of them after 2 years (Padwal, 2007). Chaput and Tremblay (2010) suggest that, while factors such as tolerability and affordability might also be reasons for stopping use, failure of Orlistat can most likely be attributed to the fact that obese patients expect to lose an average of approximately 25% of their body weight after 1 year of treatment (Foster, 1997). The efficacy of Orlistat does not meet the expectations of most patients (Chaput, 2010).

BOX 7.2 What Is "Off-Label" Use?

The FDA regulates how a medication can be advertised or promoted by the manufacturer. These regulations do not restrict a physician's ability to prescribe the medication for other conditions, in different doses, or for different lengths of time. This practice of prescribing medication for periods of time or for conditions not FDA-approved is known as off-label use. Use of more than one weight-loss medication at a time (combined drug treatment) is an example of an off-label use. Using weight-loss medications other than Orlistat for more than a short period of time is also considered off-label use (WIN, 2010).

Data from: WIN. Prescription Medications for the Treatment of Obesity. Weight-control Information Network. 2010. http://win.niddk.nih.gov/Publications/prescription.htm. Accessed March 2011.

Other Types of Medications Used for Obesity Treatment

Some categories of drugs, although not FDA-approved for the treatment of obesity, have been shown to promote weight loss in clinical studies and may be prescribed off-label. Examples of these are:

- Drugs to treat depression. While antidepressant medications are FDA-approved for the treatment of depression, their use in weight loss is an off-label use. Individuals taking these medications generally lose modest amounts of weight for up to 6 months, but they tend to regain weight later even while they are still on the drug. Bupropion (which is marketed as Amfebutamone, Wellbutrin, and Zyban) is an antidepressant and antismoking drug that produced significantly more weight loss than a placebo over a year in a randomized clinical trial. However, not enough evidence exists to recommend Bupropion as a long-term weight-loss drug (Anderson, 2002).

- Drugs to treat seizures. Two medications used to treat seizures, Topiramate and Zonisamide, have been shown to cause weight loss. Unfortunately the epilepsy drug Topiramate also produced significant side effects during several 6- to 12-month trials so the manufacturer discontinued further studies of the formula for weight loss (Glandt, 2011).

- Drugs to treat type 2 diabetes. The diabetes medication metformin has been shown to promote small amounts of weight loss in people with obesity and type 2 diabetes. Clinical trials found that metformin produced a 1- to 3-kg weight loss over an average of 2.8 years in the randomized, double blind Diabetes Prevention Program. It is not clear how this medication promotes weight loss, although people taking the drug report that they have reduced hunger and food intake (Knowler, 2002).

- Drug combinations. Little well-conducted scientific information is available about the safety or effectiveness of drug combinations for weight loss. At this time using combinations of medications for weight loss is not recommended, except as part of a research study (WIN, 2010).

Potential Benefits of Weight-Loss Medications

Weight loss with some medications may reduce a number of health risks in people who are obese. Small, sustained reductions in weight can significantly improve cardiovascular risk factors, particularly blood pressure, blood cholesterol, and triglycerides, and insulin resistance. However, at present there a few definitive studies that establish the long-term effects of weight-loss drugs on weight and health.

Individual response to weight-loss medications varies and some people experience more weight loss than others. In general, use of weight-loss medications results in an average weight loss of about 10 lb more than nondrug obesity treatments. Maximum weight loss usually occurs within 6 months of starting the medicine and then tends to level off or increase (WIN, 2010). The magnitude of weight loss may be closely linked to underlying factors that originally contributed to an individual's weight gain. If anxiety or depression drives overeating, then medication that promotes weight loss while also treating the underlying depression might be a reasonable choice (Balkon, 2011).

Potential Risks Associated with Weight-Loss Medications

Research has yet to reveal the long-term health effects of weight-loss drugs. Most studies have lasted only a year or less. In addition, research has not examined rare side effects (those occurring in less than 1 per 1,000 patients), and the optimal duration of treatment is unknown. According to the Weight-Control Information Network, a service that provides information to consumers and is sponsored by the National Institute of Diabetes and Digestive and Kidney Diseases (NIDDK), the following are potential risks of long-term weight-loss drugs to treat obesity (WIN, 2010):

- Potential for abuse or dependence. All prescription medications to treat obesity except

Orlistat are controlled substances. Physicians must follow certain restrictions when prescribing them. Abuse and dependence are not common with most appetite-suppressant medications, but they should be used with caution in patients with a history of alcohol or other drug abuse.

- Development of tolerance and weight regain. Most studies show that weight loss tends to level off after 6 months even when patients are still taking the drug. While this may be related to tolerance to the medications, the leveling off may mean that the maximum amount of weight loss that the drug can produce has been achieved. There are studies that demonstrate that, even though the weight comes back, patients receiving a weight-loss drug regain fewer pounds compared with patients in a placebo group.

- Side effects. Weight-loss drugs are used to treat a condition that affects millions of people who may be basically healthy. The possibility that side effects may outweigh benefits is a significant concern. While serious and even fatal outcomes have been reported most side effects of these drugs are mild and usually improve with continued use.

- Reluctance to make behavioral changes while using prescription medications. Weight-loss drugs are not magic pills or a quick fix for obesity. They should always be combined with a healthy eating plan and increased physical activity.

Treatment Guidelines

When a pharmacotherapeutic regimen is prescribed for obesity treatment it must be with careful consideration of risk versus benefit. The 1998 NHLBI Clinical Guidelines on the Identification, Evaluation, and Treatment of Overweight and Obesity in Adults suggest pharmacotherapy only after a patient has tried at least 6 months of diet, physical activity, and behavior therapy. Weight-loss medications are not intended for cosmetic reasons but only for people who are classified as obese or who have a BMI of 27 to 29.9 and comorbidities such as hypertension, dyslipidemia, type 2 diabetes, or sleep apnea. Other cautions set forth in the NHLBI guidelines state that, since obesity is a chronic disorder, the short-term use of drugs is not typically helpful and health professionals should include drugs only in the context of a long-term treatment strategy. Although drugs are part of the regimen, scheduled medical visits ought to be part of the treatment to monitor weight and blood parameters; discuss side effects; and answer patient concerns and questions. Treatment success is defined as at least 2-kg weight loss during the first month of drug therapy (1 lb per week), a fall more than 5% below baseline by 3 to 6 months, and remaining at this level. If these goals are not achieved, then the dose should be adjusted or the medication discontinued. The guidelines state that the use of a drug may be continued as long as it is effective and the adverse effects are manageable and there is no specification about how long a weight-loss drug should be continued (NHLBI, 1998). The ASBP obesity treatment guidelines place emphasis on health measures other than BMI citing evidence that suggests treatment based solely on BMI thresholds is inappropriate and that early, more aggressive treatment may help prevent comorbidities (Steelman, 2010). Although weight loss is an important treatment outcome, the ultimate goal of obesity management should be to improve metabolic risk factors that will reduce obesity-related morbidity and mortality. While weight loss as low as 5% of initial body weight can lead to favorable improvements in blood pressure, serum lipid concentrations, and increased insulin sensitivity, individuals who have type 2 diabetes or hypertension are the ones who have the most improvement in cardiovascular risk factors (Douketis, 2005).

Because there is a dramatic disparity between patients' expectations and realistic outcomes, an important aspect of pharmacological treatment for obesity is to help patients accept more modest weight-loss outcomes. Numerous studies have shown that obese individuals want to lose the equivalent of 25 to 35% of their initial weight and expect to do so in approximately 1 year of treatment (Foster, 1997). Dieters maintain these expectations even when they are informed that a realistic treatment goal is usually a loss of 5 to 10% of initial body weight over a 6- to 12-month period (Wadden, 2003). It is important that patients understand that there is a maximal drug effect after which weight loss plateaus. When drug therapy is discontinued, generally the weight is regained. As a result of reduced energy expenditure after weight loss more effort must be made to maintain the lower weight (Korner, 2004).

Will Insurance Cover the Cost of Weight-Loss Medication?

When considering antiobesity therapy the financial aspect should be taken into account. For example, taking Orlistat with three meals a day may cost as much as $200 a month. These expenses could become a major obstacle, especially in low-income populations. Although the situation is changing as insurers begin to recognize obesity as a chronic disease, many insurance companies will not pay for weight-loss drugs. Insurance companies may regard these drugs as cosmetic procedure exclusions and decline reimbursement. Therefore, individuals without another comorbid condition may have to pay out-of-pocket for antiobesity therapy.

Over-the-Counter (OTC) Medications for Weight Loss/Management

The FDA requires that all weight-loss OTC products have an approved Drug Facts label that educates consumers about the medication. These labels have a standard format that is intended to be easy for typical consumers to understand. Drug Facts labels include information on the product's active ingredient(s), indications and purpose, safety warnings, directions for use, and inactive ingredients, and how to contact the manufacturer. **Figure 7.2** shows how these components are listed on an OTC drug label.

Although consumers typically assume that OTC drugs on the market must be effective and safe, that has not always been the case. For instance, amphetamines were widely used for decades even though they were associated with increased cardiovascular and psychiatric disorders. They

---

BOX 7.3 **What Is the Difference Between Prescription Drugs and OTC Drugs?**

Prescription drugs are:

Prescribed by a doctor.
Bought at a pharmacy.
Prescribed for and intended to be used by one person.
Regulated by the FDA through the New Drug Application process that requires the drug sponsor to show all animal and human data as well as information about how the drug behaves in the body and how it is manufactured.

OTC drugs are:

Drugs that do NOT require a doctor's prescription.
Bought off the shelf in stores.
Regulated by the FDA through OTC drug monographs, a kind of "recipe book" that covers acceptable ingredients, doses, formulations, and labeling.

Source: FDA. Prescription Drugs and Over-the-Counter (OTC) Drugs: Questions and Answers. http://www.fda.gov/Drugs/ResourcesForYou/Consumers/QuestionsAnswers/ucm100101.htm.

---

are now restricted as controlled drugs. Another popular dieting aid was ephedra, also commonly known as Ma Huang. This shrub-like plant has been used in Chinese medicine for over 2,500 years. The active ingredient, Ephedrine, is chemically similar to amphetamines, drugs that powerfully stimulate the nervous system and heart even as they decrease appetite and increase metabolism. Ephedra has been shown to boost weight loss, and it was a popular weight-loss product until it was banned in the United States by the FDA in

FIGURE 7.2   Example of over-the-counter (OTC) drug label.

Drug Facts

Active Ingredient (in each tablet)   Purpose
Chlorpheniramine maleate 2 mg...Antihistamine

Uses temporarily relieves these symptoms due to hay fever or other upper respiratory allergies: ■ sneezing   ■ runny nose   ■ itchy, watery eyes   ■ itchy throat

Warnings
Ask a doctor before use if you have
■ glaucoma   ■ a breathing problem such as emphysema or chronic bronchitis
■ trouble urinating due to an enlarged prostate gland

Ask a doctor or pharmacist before use if you are taking tranquilizers or sedatives

When using this product
■ drowsiness may occur   ■ avoid alcoholic drinks
■ alcohol, sedatives, and tranquilizers may increase drowsiness
■ be careful when driving a motor vehicle or operating machinery
■ excitability may occur, especially in children

If pregnant or breast-feeding, ask a health professional before use.
Keep out of reach of children. In case of overdose, get medical help or contact a Poison Control Center right away.

Directions

adults and children 12 years and over	take 2 tablets every 4 to 6 hours; not more than 12 tablets in 24 hours
children 6 years to under 12 years	take 1 tablet every 4 to 6 hours; not more than 6 tablets in 24 hours
children under 6 years	ask a doctor

Other Information ■ store at 20-25°C (68-77°F)   ■ protect from excessive moisture

Inactive Ingredients D&C yellow no. 10. lactose, magnesium stearate, microcrystalline cellulose, pregelatinized starch

Courtesy of: U.S. Food and Drug Administration.

2006 due to safety concerns. There were 19,000 adverse events reported including heart attacks, strokes, or seizures. It was concluded that no dose of Ephedrine was safe and that the sale of these products in the United States was illegal. According to the FDA, there is little evidence that ephedra is effective except for short-term weight loss (NCCAM, 2006). The drug Phenylpropanolamine, used to treat nasal congestion, also reduced appetite so it was used in nonprescription diet aids for weight loss. Dexatrim, a popular appetite suppressant for over 25 years contained Phenylpropanolamine. Ultimately the drug was removed from the product line because of side effects such as increased risk for bleeding in the brain. Dexatrim products are now drug-free. Instead, they are based on a blend of botanicals as well as several vitamins and minerals and green tea extract as a common ingredient.

While some ingredients like caffeine or tea in OTC weight-loss medications slightly increase energy expenditure and may be helpful for weight control, the concentration of these ingredients is probably too small to cause weight loss in most people. Most OTC weight-loss products come with instructions that point out that the diet aid works best when combined with a sensible meal plan and regular exercise. The truth is that most people could probably achieve the same results with diet and exercise alone.

Dietary Supplement Therapies for Weight Loss

A frequent question among people who are dieting is: What herbs or supplements should I take to lose weight? A survey indicated that more than a quarter of American women trying to lose weight had tried over-the-counter weight-loss supplements (Blanck, 2007). Supplements are attractive because they are often marketed as "natural," which may be interpreted as an assurance of safety. It is possible that the choice to supplement a diet with particular botanicals, vitamins, minerals, or other products may be a sensible decision that improves well being and vitality. However, it is confusing to sift through the questionable claims to find accurate information about supplements and their side effects or benefits.

Congress defined the term *dietary supplement* in the Dietary Supplement Health and Education Act (DSHEA) of 1994 as a product taken by mouth that contains a dietary ingredient intended to supplement the diet. The dietary ingredients in these products may include vitamins, minerals, herbs or other botanicals, amino acids, and substances such as enzymes, organ tissues, glandulars, and metabolites (USDA, 1995). According to the DSHEA, dietary supplements cannot legally claim to prevent, mitigate, treat, or cure a specific disease. Nevertheless misleading weight-loss claims are common. Producers promise a wide variety of

ways to reduce fat including increasing energy expenditure, increasing satiety, increasing fat oxidation, and blocking dietary fat absorption.

Supplements Regulation and FDA Oversight

As a result of the DSHEA dietary supplements are defined and regulated as foods, not drugs. Dietary supplements can be marketed without FDA approval and without any scientific evidence to substantiate safety or efficacy. The manufacturer is responsible for ensuring that its products are safe before they are marketed. Furthermore, dietary supplement producers are not required by law to record, investigate, or notify the FDA about any reports of adverse events that may be related to the use of their products. The FDA can take action to remove the product from the market only after a supplement has been shown to be unsafe for consumers (Larsen, 2003).

An assessment of consumer knowledge and beliefs about dietary supplements by Pillitteri and colleagues (2008) demonstrated that consumers know very little about the regulation, safety, and efficacy of dietary supplements. Both users and nonusers agreed that dietary supplements are effective in helping people to lose weight. Substantial numbers believed that the FDA reviews and approves supplements despite statements on supplement packages indicating that the FDA has not reviewed the products.

Dietary supplements are widely used for many reasons. They may appeal to those who want more autonomy over the decisions related to their health. Others may choose dietary supplements for help losing weight as a result of dissatisfaction with conventional weight-loss treatments (Astin, 1998). Supplements are easily available without a prescription that requires a doctor visit. Research suggests that few patients tell their doctor about supplement use. A 2007 study of weight-loss supplement users found that only 30% told their healthcare professionals that they were taking these products (Blanck, 2007). Healthcare providers should inquire about dietary supplement use by their patients and take the opportunity to discuss misconceptions about safety and efficacy of supplements and the risk for adverse events as some of these products can interact with prescription medications.

While some supplement suppliers allege that mainstream scientists try to suppress information about miraculous alternative products, there is much ongoing conventional research to study the benefits and the risks of dietary supplements. The National Center for Complementary and Alternative Medicine (NCCAM), an agency of the federal government, is devoted to rigorous scientific investigation of herbs and supplements. To get information on any of thousands of studies from NCCAM see the Resources section in this chapter.

How Is Advertising of Weight-Loss Products Regulated?

In September 2002, the Federal Trade Commission (FTC) released a report titled *Weight Loss Advertising: An Analysis of Current Trends*. This report indicated that the use of false and misleading claims in weight-loss advertising was widespread (USFTC, 2002). The commission found that 55% of weight-loss ads made claims that were misleading, lacked proof, or were obviously false. Researchers examined 300 weight-loss advertisements taken from television, radio, the Internet, newspapers, magazines, e-mail, and direct mail. The FTC study provided numerous examples of false or exaggerated claims and reported about specific weight-loss supplements that lacked safety warnings and could be dangerous.

Red Flag Campaign

The FTC launched a Red Flag Campaign to help media voluntarily identify and "red flag" ads with fraudulent weight-loss claims and to screen out ads containing claims that are too good to be true (USFTC, 2002). The following claims are those that should alert the public and the media that an advertisement should be met with skepticism. Red Flags are claims that a product can:

- Cause weight loss of 2 lb or more a week for a month or more without dieting or exercise.
- Cause substantial weight loss no matter what or how much the consumer eats.

- Cause permanent weight loss (even when the consumer stops using the product).
- Block the absorption of fat or calories to enable consumers to lose substantial weight.
- Safely enable consumers to lose more than 3 lb per week for more than 4 weeks.
- Cause substantial weight loss for all users.
- Bring about weight loss that exceeds what is physiologically possible under normal circumstances, for example, losing 120 lb in 7 weeks.

A list of products identified by the FTC as examples of fraudulent weight-loss products can be found on the FTC website.

Because there is a wide array of dietary supplements that are promoted and heavily advertised for weight loss, it is difficult for most dieters to decide which supplement to use. There are dozens of products to choose from and examples of supplements sold for weight loss range from botanicals including green tea, bitter orange, or yerba mate; hormones such as human chorionic gonadotropin (hCG); the amino acid 5-hydroxytryptophan (5-HTP); the fatty acid conjugated linoleic acid (CLA); the mineral chromium; to glucomannan fiber supplements. To make sense of whether any of these are safe and actually work for reliable weight management, scientifically based information about botanicals and supplements can be found on websites managed by the United States Office of Dietary Supplements (ODS), the National Center for Complementary and Alternative Medicine (NCCAM), or the Natural Medicines Comprehensive Database. These websites are listed in the Resources section of this chapter.

Summary

Medication for treating obesity, if prescribed and monitored by a physician, may be a beneficial adjunct to a weight-loss regimen when combined with lifestyle, behavioral, and dietary modifications. Pharmacotherapy as a strategy for obesity management remains controversial, and the potential risks of drug interventions must be weighed against the benefits. The effect of medication is modest and is often limited by side effects. Weight loss lasts only as long as the drug is being taken as most weight is regained as soon as treatment is stopped. Although several pharmaceuticals have been shown to be valuable in short-term and long-term therapy, several products have voluntarily been removed from the United States marketplace because of serious or fatal side effects.

Nonprescription drug and dietary supplement use is common among individuals who want to lose weight. However, consumers have misconceptions about the safety, efficacy, and regulation of these products. The proliferation of dietary supplements on the market, the ease of obtaining these products, and extreme claims of effectiveness make it difficult to assess their safety and efficacy. Healthcare providers and consumers should look to credible sources of information when selecting pharmaceuticals and supplements for weight control.

Critical Thinking Questions

Question: Discuss the idea that the FDA and other regulatory agencies hold antiobesity drugs to higher standards than drugs for other serious medical conditions. What are the individual and population health consequences?

Question: Most of the drugs approved for obesity have been approved by the FDA for short-term use only. The American Society of Bariatric Physicians regards weight-loss medications as a treatment that can be used as needed, and the NHLBI guidelines state there is no specification about how long a weight-loss drug should be continued. What explanations can you give for the divergence of opinion among these groups?

Question: What kinds of weight-loss drugs or supplements have you seen in the martketplace? Check the labels to see if there is information about the safety and efficacy of the products.

Question: Apply the weight-loss supplement Red Flag criteria to some product advertisements that are currently in the media.

Resources

alli

http://www.myalli.com

The site provides information about side effects, drug interactions, and usage recommendations for the drug alli.

Dietary Supplement Labeling.

http://www.fda.gov/Food/DietarySupplements/default.htm

FDA Drug Questions and Answers Website.

http://www.fda.gov/Drugs/ResourcesForYou/default.htm

Fraudulent Weight-Loss Products.

http://www.fda.gov/Drugs/DrugSafety/default.htm

http://www.ftc.gov/opa/2007/01/weightloss.shtm

National Center for Complementary and Alternative Medicine (NCCAM), National Institutes of Health, Health Topics A–Z.

http://nccam.nih.gov/health/atoz.htm

NCCAM is the federal government's lead agency for scientific research on the diverse medical and healthcare systems, practices, and products that are not generally considered part of conventional medicine.

Natural Medicines Comprehensive Database: Scientific Clinical Information on Complementary, Alternative, and Integrative Therapies.

http://naturaldatabase.therapeuticresearch.com

Office of Dietary Supplements.

http://ods.od.nih.gov/factsheets/botanicalbackground.asp

This site contains general information on botanicals and their use as dietary supplements.

References

Anderson JW, Greenway FL, Fujioka K, Gadde KM, McKenney J, O'Neil PM. Bupropion SR enhances weight loss: a 48-week double-blind, placebo-controlled trial. *Obes Res.* Jul 2002;10(7):633–641.

ASBP. American Society of Bariatric Physicians. Overweight and Obesity Evaluation and Management. 2009; http://www.asbp.org/resources. Accessed April 10, 2011.

Astin JA. Why patients use alternative medicine: results of a national study. *JAMA.* May 20 1998;279(19): 1548–1553.

Balkon N, Balkon C, Zitkus BS. Overweight and obesity: pharmacotherapeutic considerations. *J Am Acad Nurse Pract.* Feb 2011;23(2):61–66.

Blanck HM, Serdula MK, Gillespie C, et al. Use of nonprescription dietary supplements for weight loss is common among Americans. *J Am Diet Assoc.* Mar 2007;107(3):441–447.

Bolen SD, Clark JM, Richards TM, Shore AD, Goodwin SM, Weiner JP. Trends in and patterns of obesity reduction medication use in an insured cohort. *Obesity (Silver Spring).* Jan 2010;18(1): 206–209.

Cercato C, Roizenblatt VA, Leanca CC, et al. A randomized double-blind placebo-controlled study of the long-term efficacy and safety of diethylpropion in the treatment of obese subjects. *Int J Obes (Lond).* Aug 2009;33(8):857–865.

Chaput JP, Tremblay A. Well-being of obese individuals: therapeutic perspectives. *Future Med Chem.* Dec 2010;2(12):1729–1733.

Connolly HM, Crary JL, McGoon MD, et al. Valvular heart disease associated with fenfluramine-phentermine. *N Engl J Med.* Aug 28 1997;337(9):581–588.

Davidson MH, Hauptman J, DiGirolamo M, et al. Weight control and risk factor reduction in obese subjects treated for 2 years with orlistat: a randomized controlled trial. *JAMA.* Jan 20 1999;281(3):235–242.

Douketis JD, Macie C, Thabane L, Williamson DF. Systematic review of long-term weight loss studies in obese adults: clinical significance and applicability to clinical practice. *Int J Obes (Lond).* Oct 2005; 29(10):1153–1167.

FDA. Guidance for Industry Developing Products for Weight Management. 2007; http://www.fda.gov/downloads/Drugs/GuidanceCompliance Regulatory Information /Guidances/ucm071612.pdf. Accessed April 19, 2011.

Foster GD, Wadden TA, Vogt RA, Brewer G. What is a reasonable weight loss? Patients' expectations and evaluations of obesity treatment outcomes. *J Consult Clin Psychol.* Feb 1997;65(1):79–85.

Glandt M, Raz I. Present and future: pharmacologic treatment of obesity. *J Obes.* 2011:636181.

Hendricks EJ, Greenway FL, Westman EC, Gupta AK. Blood pressure and heart rate effects, weight loss and maintenance during long-term phentermine pharmacotherapy for obesity. *Obesity (Silver Spring).* Dec 2011;19(12):2351-2360.

Hendricks EJ, Rothman RB, Greenway FL. How physician obesity specialists use drugs to treat obesity. *Obesity (Silver Spring).* Sep 2009;17(9):1730–1735.

James WP, Caterson ID, Coutinho W, et al. Effect of sibutramine on cardiovascular outcomes in overweight and obese subjects. *N Engl J Med.* Sep 2 2010; 363(10):905–917.

Jeffery RW, Drewnowski A, Epstein LH, et al. Long-term maintenance of weight loss: current status. *Health Psychol.* Jan 2000;19(1 Suppl):5–16.

Knowler WC, Barrett-Connor E, Fowler SE, et al. Reduction in the incidence of type 2 diabetes with lifestyle intervention or metformin. *N Engl J Med.* Feb 7 2002;346(6):393–403.

Korner J, Aronne LJ. Pharmacological approaches to weight reduction: therapeutic targets. *J Clin Endocrinol Metab.* Jun 2004;89(6):2616–2621.

Larsen LL, Berry JA. The regulation of dietary supplements. *J Am Acad Nurse Pract.* Sep 2003;15(9):410–414.

Leite CE, Mocelin CA, Petersen GO, Leal MB, Thiesen FV. Rimonabant: an antagonist drug of the endocannabinoid system for the treatment of obesity. *Pharmacol Rep.* Mar–Apr 2009;61(2):217–224.

Munro JF, MacCuish AC, Wilson EM, Duncan LJ. Comparison of continuous and intermittent anorectic therapy in obesity. *Br Med J.* Feb 10 1968;1(5588): 352–354.

NCCAM. National Center for Complementary and Alternative Medicine. Ephedra, 2006; http://nccam.nih .gov/health/ephedra/. Accessed December 2010.

NHLBI. National Heart, Lung, and Blood Institute. Clinical guidelines on the identification, evaluation, and treatment of overweight and obesity in adults: executive summary. Vol. No. 98-4083. Bethesda, MD: National Institutes of Health; 1998.

Padwal R, Kezouh A, Levine M, Etminan M. Long-term persistence with orlistat and sibutramine in a population-based cohort. *Int J Obes (Lond).* Oct 2007;31(10):1567–1570.

Pillitteri JL, Shiffman S, Rohay JM, Harkins AM, Burton SL, Wadden TA. Use of dietary supplements for weight loss in the United States: results of a national survey. *Obesity (Silver Spring).* Apr 2008;16(4): 790–796.

Robinson JR, Niswender KD. What are the risks and the benefits of current and emerging weight-loss medications? *Curr Diab Rep.* Oct 2009;9(5):368–375.

Rucker D, Padwal R, Li SK, Curioni C, Lau DC. Long term pharmacotherapy for obesity and overweight: updated meta-analysis. *BMJ.* Dec 8 2007;335(7631): 1194–1199.

Sargent BJ, Moore NA. New central targets for the treatment of obesity. *Br J Clin Pharmacol.* Dec 2009;68(6): 852–860.

Stafford RS, Radley DC. National trends in antiobesity medication use. *Arch Intern Med.* May 12 2003;163(9): 1046–1050.

Steelman GM, Westman EC. *Obesity: Evaluation and Treatment Essentials.* New York: Informa Healthcare; 2010.

USDA. U.S. Food and Drug Administration. Dietary Supplement Health and Education Act of 1994. College Park, MD: U.S. Food and Drug Administration. Center for Food Safety and Applied Nutrition; 1995.

USFTC. *Weight-Loss Advertising: An Analysis of Current Trends.* Washington, DC: U.S. Federal Trade Commission; 2002.

Wadden TA, Womble LG, Sarwer DB, Berkowitz RI, Clark VL, Foster GD. Great expectations: "I'm losing 25% of my weight no matter what you say." *J Consult Clin Psychol.* Dec 2003;71(6):1084–1089.

WIN. Prescription Medications for the Treatment of Obesity. Weight-control Information Network. 2010; http://win.niddk.nih.gov/Publications/prescription.htm. Accessed March 2011.

CHAPTER 8

SURGICAL OPTIONS FOR OBESITY

READER OBJECTIVES

- Discuss historic and current trends in bariatric surgery
- Identify indications and eligibility criteria for weight-loss surgery
- Compare preparation procedures, follow-up, and results for gastric bypass and gastric banding surgeries
- Summarize the theories about how the surgeries contribute to excess weight loss and metabolic benefits
- List risks associated with obesity surgeries
- Discuss how bariatric surgery success is defined
- Explain the role of insurance companies in covering the costs of obesity surgeries
- Describe why jaw wiring and liposuction are ineffective for long-term weight loss and body fat reduction

CHAPTER OUTLINE

Surgery for Severe Obesity

Although the increasing incidence of obesity is undoubtedly due to an imbalance of energy intake and energy output, lack of an effective treatment for obesity is also a significant contributor to this serious public health problem. Long-term weight loss is difficult to achieve with diet, exercise, or pharmacotherapy. Most **bariatric** surgery patients have already experienced numerous attempts to achieve a sustained weight loss by using nonsurgical treatment options. To date, bariatric surgery has been shown to be the only intervention to induce significant weight loss in people with severe obesity and to meaningfully improve chronic health conditions, survival, and quality of life (Adams, 2007; Sjostrom, 2007).

History

In 1954, Drs. Arnold Kremen and John Linner at the University of Minnesota were studying food absorption in dogs. They discovered that the animals lost weight after they underwent operations that bypassed a large part of their intestinal tract (Kremen, 1954). This surgery was subsequently successfully performed on one of Dr. Linner's human patients who asked him to use the technique on her in the hopes that she, too, could lose weight. With a growing number of obese patients seeking alternatives to diets, medical professionals began to recognize bariatric surgery as a possible treatment for obesity. Initially, there were high rates of complications with some of the operations, and the procedure remained controversial until the National Institutes of Health (NIH) convened a consensus conference on surgery for obesity in 1991. A panel of experts concluded that various surgical alterations of the digestive system appeared to reduce excess body fat in many people without severe side effects. They approved bariatric surgery as an effective option for severely obese individuals who had failed more moderate weight-reduction strategies (NIH, 1991).

Incidence

Bariatric surgery has gained in acceptance and popularity, as evidenced by substantial increases in the procedure. In 1999 singer Carnie Wilson had gastric bypass surgery and allowed the actual procedure to be broadcast live over the Internet; it was viewed by more than 500,000 people. Since that time, the number of bariatric surgeries increased dramatically from 16,000 to almost 220,000 in 2009 (ASMBS, 2010). The majority of patients is female, between 40 and 64 years of age, with higher socioeconomic status, and privately insured (Santry, 2007). The increase in bariatric surgery numbers nationwide has probably been fueled by a combination of increasing public awareness and demand along with new minimally invasive techniques and the continuing failure of nonsurgical treatments to provide effective sustained weight loss. The future outlook is for the number of bariatric surgeries to continue to grow. It is estimated that 15 million people in the United States have extreme obesity, and even with the large number of procedures currently performed, less than 1% of eligible individuals undergo bariatric surgery (ASMBS, 2010).

Indications

The 1998 NHLBI obesity clinical guidelines for adults set the patient selection criterion for obesity surgery as a BMI of 40 or more or a BMI between 35 and 40 accompanied by high-risk obesity comorbidities such as type 2 diabetes, hypertension, sleep apnea, asthma, or osteoarthritis of weight-bearing joints. Surgery eligibility also extends to those with a BMI of at least 35 who have physical alterations that limit everyday life activities and to individuals who have not been able to achieve a satisfactory weight through diet, exercise, and medication. Surgery is recommended only for patients who have an acceptable risk for surgery, are well-informed, motivated, and able to participate in treatment and long-term follow-up. Patients who choose surgery will require lifelong medical care and should work with a multidisciplinary team including medical, nutritional, and behavioral specialists (NHLBI, 1998). While the NIH guidelines have remained unchanged since 1991, newer criteria for adults are being evaluated. The current BMI standard may no longer be appropriate because there is increasing evidence that bariatric surgery can reverse comorbidities such as type 2 diabetes even in patients with a BMI of less than 30 (Pories, 2010). Walter Pories, one of the pioneers in bariatric surgery, suggests that applying an adjusted BMI, which takes into account sex, race, age, fitness, or body fat composition, would be a more realistic criterion.

Age Limits

There are no specific age limits for bariatric surgery. For older adults age guidelines from the American Society for Metabolic & Bariatric Surgery (ASMBS) suggest that patients eligible for surgery should be 18 to 65 years old. Individuals outside that age range who undergo surgery should have significant health conditions related to obesity, and the expectation of improved life expectancy or quality of life should outweigh the risk of surgery (Mechanick, 2008). The NHLBI clinical guidelines summarized available data regarding any type of weight reduction after age 65 and recommended:

> A clinical decision to forgo obesity treatment in an older adult should be guided by an evaluation of the potential benefits of weight reduction for day-to-day functioning and reduction of the risk of future cardiovascular events, as well as the patient's motivation for weight reduction. (NHLBI, 1998)

An increasing number of young people with a BMI of greater than 40 and severe comorbidities, such as type 2 diabetes, are undergoing bariatric surgery. Supporting research shows bariatric surgery in adolescents is associated with weight loss, reducing the risks associated with metabolic disorders, and improved self-image and socialization (Lawson, 2006; Xanthakos, 2008). As long-term data including information on malabsorption of critical nutrients and effects on maturation are unknown, experts advise that surgical therapy should be reserved for full-grown adolescents with treatment by experienced multidisciplinary teams who can provide comprehensive medical and psychological care (Livingston, 2010b). Bariatric procedures are generally contraindicated for pre-adolescent age groups, as long-term health effects, durability of the weight loss, and life expectancy for teens who undergo operations remain largely unknown. In 2007 the NIH launched a study to evaluate the benefits and risks of bariatric surgery in adolescents. The Teen Longitudinal Assessment of Bariatric Surgery (Teen-LABS) study was designed to help determine if surgery is an appropriate treatment option for extremely overweight teens. The researchers aim to enroll 200 adolescents who are scheduled for bariatric surgery so their outcomes can be compared to 200 adults who have had bariatric surgery. For more information about Teen-LABS, see the website listed in the Resources section of this chapter.

Though surgery may be a promising treatment for extreme obesity in youth, the acceptability of bariatric surgical interventions for obese children and adolescents remains a topic of controversy among patients, healthcare practitioners, researchers, policymakers, and the general public. An example of the disagreement on this subject is revealed in a study about physicians' attitudes on referring obese adolescents for bariatric surgery. In this group, 48% of the participating physicians indicated that they would never refer an obese adolescent for a bariatric operation, and 46% indicated that the minimum age at which they would make a referral was 18 years (Woolford, 2010).

Contraindications

Currently, a consensus does not exist on the possible contraindications to bariatric surgery. Suggested contraindications would include an extremely high operative risk, such as severe cardiovascular disease. To help avoid adverse postoperative outcomes, patients are also screened for severe depression, untreated mental illnesses, active substance abuse, or **binge eating disorders**. Patients who cannot comprehend the nature of the surgical intervention and the lifelong measures required to maintain health, should not be offered this procedure (Mechanick, 2008).

Before Surgery

Bariatric surgery may be the next step for people who remain severely obese after trying nonsurgical approaches, especially if they have an obesity-related disease. Surgery to produce weight loss is a serious undertaking and anyone thinking about undergoing this type of operation should understand what it involves. Responding to the questionnaire "Is surgery for you?" from the Weight-control Information Network (WIN) may help an individual decide whether weight-loss surgery is the right choice.

BOX 8.1   Weight-control Information Network: Is Surgery for You?

Are you:

- Unlikely to lose weight or keep it off over the long term with nonsurgical measures?
- Well informed about the surgical procedure and the effects of treatment?
- Determined to lose weight and improve your health?
- Aware of how your life may change after the operation (adjustment to the side effects of the operation, including the need to chew food well and inability to eat large meals)?
- Aware of the potential risk for serious complications, dietary restrictions, and occasional failures?
- Committed to lifelong healthy eating and physical activity habits, medical follow-up, and vitamin/mineral supplementation?

Remember: There are no guarantees that any method, including surgery, will produce and maintain weight loss. Success is possible only with maximum cooperation and commitment to behavioral change and medical follow-up—and this cooperation and commitment must be carried out for the rest of your life.

Reproduced from: WIN. Bariatric Surgery for Severe Obesity. Weight-control Information Network, 2009. http://win.niddk.nih.gov/publications/gastric.htm

---

Because not everyone who wants gastric bypass is psychologically or medically ready for the surgical procedure, an extensive screening process is required. A team of professionals, including physicians, dietitians, psychologists, and surgeons, evaluate aspects of health that would be expected to improve after surgery, as well as what preexisting conditions might increase **perioperative** risk. Surgery is recommended only when the perceived benefits of surgery outweigh the predicted risks. To improve surgical success and to decrease the chance of weight regain later, preventive strategies should be acquired and practiced before the surgery. The patient's relationship with food must be thoroughly explored, as there are many factors that contribute to overeating. Individuals who do not learn to manage emotional contributors (eating in response to sadness or joy, eating to comfort or to alleviate stress) prior to surgery are at high risk of weight regain.

Weight Loss Before Surgery

A controversial issue among bariatric programs and health insurance companies in the United States is whether or not patients should be required to lose weight before bariatric surgery. In a randomized study of patients undergoing gastric bypass surgery preoperative weight loss of 10% was associated with improved loss over 6 months but not with long-term weight loss (Alami, 2007). Another study found that mandated preoperative weight loss did not improve postoperative weight loss, and it was associated with increased dropout rates before gastric bypass surgery (Jamal, 2006). Individuals who seek bariatric surgery usually report an extensive dieting history, which calls into question the value of mandated preoperative weight loss. While the effect on eventual weight loss is not clear, there may be a functional benefit of preoperative weight loss as shown by a study in which at least 2 weeks of a very-low-calorie diet substantially reduced liver size and thereby potentially allowed for better surgical manipulation (Colles, 2006). Patients who lose about 10% of their excess body weight in the few weeks prior to surgery are less likely to suffer from surgical complications. They have shorter operative time and hospital stays and reduced blood loss compared to those who do not lose weight prior to surgery (Still, 2007). The most realistic preoperative weight-loss requirements should be based on reducing risk during surgery and the patient's history of previous weight-loss interventions.

Categories of Procedures

Malabsorptive Versus Restrictive

Bariatric surgeries are categorized as malabsorptive, restrictive, or a combination of the two. Restrictive surgeries primarily reduce the size of the stomach thus restricting the amount of food that can be consumed at one time. Malabsorptive procedures may also reduce the size of the stomach but mainly aim to cause nutrient malabsorption through bypass of a portion of the small intestine with the result that food is incompletely digested and absorbed. **Figure 8.1** shows how restrictive and mixed surgeries impact the stomach and intestinal tract.

Open Versus Laparoscopic

Surgical techniques may be open or **laparoscopic**. The open procedure involves a single incision that provides the surgeon access to the abdominal cavity. Open gastric bypass, once used commonly for bariatric surgery, now accounts for only 3% of the procedures (Livingston, 2010a). Because laparoscopic procedures were introduced to bariatric surgery in the early 1990s they were not included in the 1991 NIH Consensus Conference Statement. By 2003, nearly two-thirds of bariatric procedures worldwide were performed laparoscopically (Buchwald, 2005). In laparoscopic surgery, a small video camera is inserted into the abdomen allowing the surgeon to conduct and view the procedure on a video monitor. Both camera and surgical instruments are inserted through small incisions made in the abdominal wall. Laparoscopic surgery requires smaller incisions, less postoperative pain, a briefer hospital stay, and more rapid postoperative recovery with fewer complications. Not all patients are suitable for laparoscopy. Those who are extremely obese or who have had previous abdominal surgery may require the open technique (Mechanick, 2008).

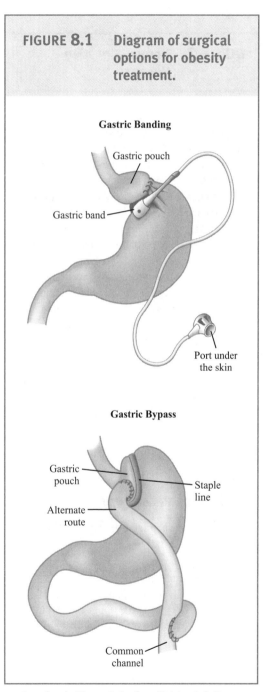

FIGURE 8.1   Diagram of surgical options for obesity treatment.

Gastric Banding

Gastric pouch

Gastric band

Port under the skin

Gastric Bypass

Gastric pouch

Staple line

Alternate route

Common channel

BOX 8.2   Normal Digestion Process

In normal digestion, food is propelled along the digestive tract where digestive juices and enzymes digest and absorb calories and nutrients. After food is swallowed it moves down the esophagus to the stomach, a pouch that can hold about 3 pints of food at a time. Stomach contents move into the duodenum, the first segment of the 20-foot-long small intestine where most of the iron and calcium in the food is absorbed. The jejunum and ileum, the remaining two segments of the small intestine, complete the absorption of almost all calories and nutrients. The food particles that cannot be digested in the small intestine are stored in the large intestine until eliminated.

Reproduced from: WIN. Bariatric Surgery for Severe Obesity. Weight-control Information Network, 2009. http://win.niddk.nih.gov/publications/gastric.htm.

Gastric Bypass Surgery

Gastric bypass surgery description (ASMBS, 2010)

- The stomach is reduced from size of football to size of golf ball.
- The stomach is attached to middle of small intestine, bypassing the upper section (duodenum and jejunum) so absorption of energy is limited.
- The surgery takes about 4 hours.
- It can be performed by both open and laparoscopic techniques.
- The hospital stay generally lasts from 3 to 5 days.

The Roux-en-Y gastric bypass, a well-known procedure, is often simply referred to as gastric bypass (GBP). See **Figure 8.2** to review the general layout of the digestive tract that is modified during GBP. During the procedure a very small section of the stomach is separated from the total to make a new mini-stomach. The resulting pouch can hold about an ounce of food. This pouch is then connected to a lower section of the small intestine, bypassing the upper part where most active digestion takes place so absorption of nutrients is greatly reduced. The extent of the bypass of the intestinal tract determines the degree of macronutrient malabsorption. Weight loss is due to both reduced food intake and reduced absorption of calories from that food. The surgery can result in loss of about 55 to 65% of excess body weight (WIN, 2009).

Treatment does not end with the surgical procedure. All bariatric surgery patients need careful medical follow-up to prevent complications, manage obesity-related health problems, and prevent weight regain. Although there are no specific dietary guidelines after bariatric surgery, patients are generally advised to follow a diet that begins with liquids only, then moves to ground up or soft foods, and finally progresses to regular foods. During the first week, meals are limited to no more than about 2 oz or about one-quarter cup per serving, four to six times per day. At 2 months postoperatively, patients can eat approximately 1 cup of food per meal. Patients are instructed on new eating patterns that avoid foods that are high in fat and sugars and include high-protein foods, as well as encourage consuming several small meals during the day, thorough chewing, and drinking liquids only between meals. View the AACE/TOS/ASMBS Guidelines listed in the Resources section of this chapter and Figure 3 in the Kulick (2010) citation in the References section for details about the postoperative diet progressions.

Complications and Risks of Gastric Bypass Surgery

As with any major surgery, bariatric procedures are not without significant risks. Early complications associated with the surgical procedure itself may be as high as 10% or more and include such events as gastrointestinal tract leakage, bowel

FIGURE **8.2**   Diagram of digestive tract.

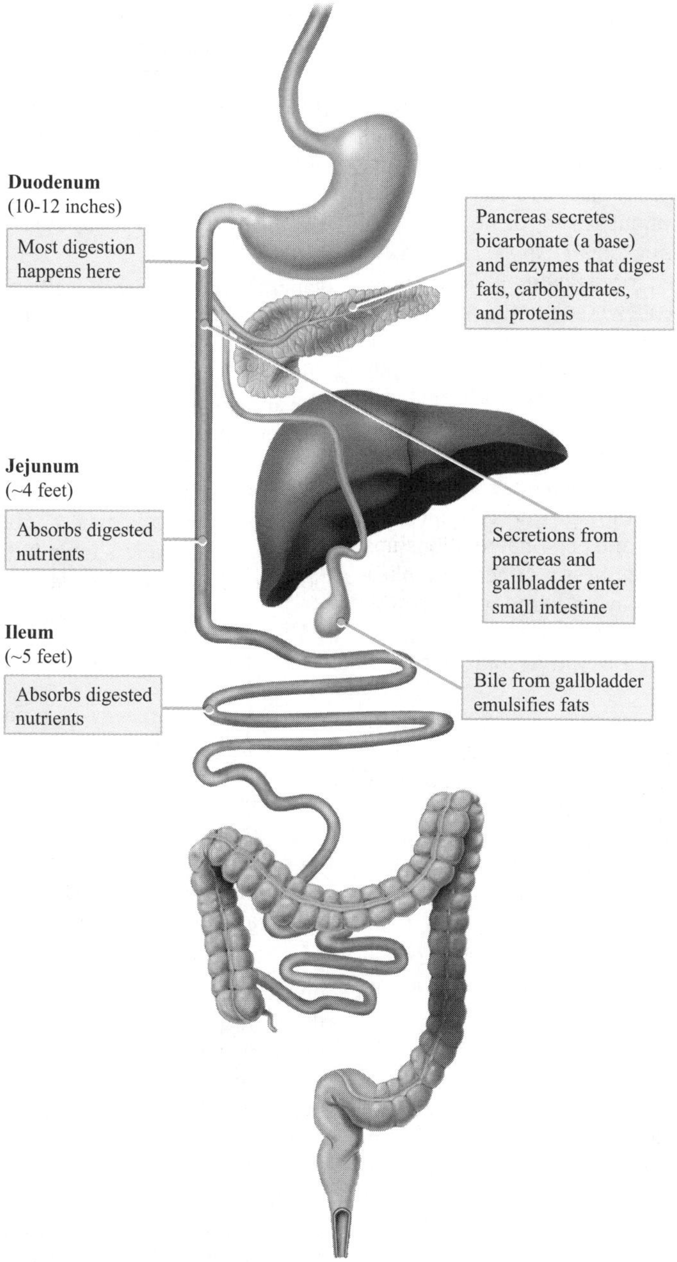

Duodenum
(10-12 inches)

Most digestion
happens here

Jejunum
(~4 feet)

Absorbs digested
nutrients

Ileum
(~5 feet)

Absorbs digested
nutrients

Pancreas secretes
bicarbonate (a base)
and enzymes that digest
fats, carbohydrates,
and proteins

Secretions from
pancreas and
gallbladder enter
small intestine

Bile from gallbladder
emulsifies fats

obstruction, bleeding, infections, complications from anesthesia, or death. Risk of death from bariatric surgery when performed by skilled surgeons is about 0.1% (ASMBS, 2010). In theory GBP can be reversed, though this is rarely done. Examples of complications necessitating surgical reversal include severe malnutrition, organ failure, or psychiatric emergencies (Mechanick, 2008).

Complications that occur later can range from infection to metabolic and emotional disturbances and malnutrition. The risk of nutritional deficiencies is a serious concern after this surgery, which involves bypassing about 1.5 m, or about 5 ft, of small intestine so it is no longer exposed to food and the enzymes required for digesting it. Deficiencies may be seen in patients who do not consume adequate protein or take their prescribed vitamins and minerals. If malnutrition is not addressed promptly, conditions such as anemia, osteoporosis, pellagra, beriberi, and kwashiorkor may occur along with permanent damage to the nervous system (WIN, 2009). Some patients may also require professional support to help them through the postoperative changes in body image and personal relationships. More information about obesity surgery complications and treatments may be found in the AACE/TOS/ASMBS Guidelines (to review these guidelines, see website listed in the Resources section of this chapter).

About 10% of patients who undergo bariatric surgery may have unsatisfactory weight loss or regain much of the weight they lose. In most patients weight loss generally levels off in 1 to 2 years, and a regain of up to 20 lb from the weight-loss low point is common (Buchwald, 2005). Behaviors such as frequent snacking on high-calorie foods, lack of exercise, or mechanical problems that may occur after the surgery, such as a stretched pouch, may also contribute to inadequate weight loss (WIN, 2009).

Centers of Excellence

Surgeon skill and bariatric surgery volume at a medical center are important factors in reducing surgical risks and complications. Compared with centers that had fewer than 50 cases per year, high-volume centers with more than 100 cases had lower mortality, shorter length of stay, fewer complications, and lower costs (Nguyen, 2004). The ASMBS and the American College of Surgeons (ACS) have established "Centers of Excellence" and certification programs in an effort to identify the best and safest practices by tracking outcomes, defining clinical criteria, enhancing the quality of care, and improving patient access to the bariatric surgeries. Many insurers, including Medicare, provide coverage for bariatric surgery only if it is performed at a medical center designated a Center of Excellence.

Benefits/Outcomes of Gastric Bypass Surgery

Patients who undergo GBP typically experience rapid weight loss and continue to do so for 12 to 18 months following surgery. They may maintain 50 to 60% of their weight loss 10 to 14 years after obesity surgery (Sjostrom, 2007). Research studies have shown that malabsorptive and restrictive procedures can improve or resolve more than 30 obesity-related conditions. According to a review of studies of more than 22,000 surgery patients, improvements were shown in the following metabolic conditions (Buchwald, 2004):

- Type 2 diabetes remission occurred in 76.8% of patients and significantly improved in 86% of patients.
- Hypertension was eliminated in 62% of patients and significantly improved in 79% of patients.
- High cholesterol was reduced in more than 70% of patients.
- Sleep apnea was eliminated in 86% of patients.
- Joint disease, asthma, and infertility were also dramatically improved or resolved.

As compared to those who do not have surgery individuals who have GBP procedures may increase their lifespan with a reduced risk of premature death of 30 to 40% (Christou, 2004).

For many individuals, weight loss results in purely mechanical benefits such as less weight bearing on joints that reduces arthritis symptoms or decreased fatty tissue around the chest and neck, which can relieve breathing obstruction and sleep apnea. There are also important metabolic changes related to gastric surgery, which are independent of weight loss, that act by altering gut hormones (Nagle 2010). Many patients with type 2 diabetes experience complete remission within days of obesity surgery, long before significant weight comes off. Altered gut hormones may be responsible for type 2 diabetes resolution in up to 95% of patients who undergo malabsorptive procedures (Buchwald, 2009). Because there is compelling evidence that shows bariatric surgery may be among the most effective treatments for metabolic diseases and conditions including type 2 diabetes, hypertension, and abnormal cholesterol levels, the procedures are now often referred to as metabolic and bariatric surgery (ASMBS, 2010). Metabolic surgery is defined as the treatment of metabolic derangements by way of alterations in the gut anatomy. This has led to new thinking that the surgery is not only effective for weight reduction but may also be appropriate for individuals with type 2 diabetes who are at normal weight or only slightly overweight.

Laparoscopic Adjustable Gastric Banding

In 1993, adjustable gastric banding was introduced. It was a new type of surgery, with the advantages of a minimally invasive adjustability and complete reversibility (Catona, 1993). The surgery is most often done with laparoscopy; therefore, it is called laparoscopic adjustable gastric banding or LAGB. In this purely restrictive procedure, an adjustable band is placed around the upper part of the stomach, creating a small pouch that holds only about 1 to 2 Tbsp of food. The smaller stomach fills up with food quickly, produces a sensation of fullness, and reduces food intake. The food passes slowly into the main part of the stomach through a small opening, or **stoma**, and then on to the rest of the digestive system. This operation leaves the main part of the digestive system unchanged. The band is actually a balloon filled with saline solution that keeps the opening from expanding and is designed to stay in place indefinitely. Adding or removing saline through an access port can adjust the size of the pouch opening. Adjustment of the band is an essential part of LAGB therapy. Adjustments may be performed up

to six times per year and are essential for successful outcomes (Buchwald, 2005).

Outcomes Associated with Gastric Banding

Gastric banding typically produces a 40 to 50% loss of excess body weight in the 2 years after surgery (WIN, 2009). Patients who have gastric banding lose less weight than those who have malabsorptive procedures and degree of weight reduction depends on following a strict diet. For some patients, failure to achieve optimal weight loss is associated with consumption of calorically dense liquids that can readily pass through the stoma without producing a sense of fullness (Mechanick, 2008). Mortality associated with LAGB when performed by skilled surgeons is about 0.1%. Operative morbidity is about 5% (Buchwald, 2005). Long-term complications of LAGB include obstruction of the stoma, stretching of the gastric pouch, infection, and access port problems. Laparoscopic adjustable gastric banding can be completely reversed with removal of the band. For more details on types of obesity surgery, see the website listed under Bariatric Surgery for Severe Obesity: What Are the Surgical Options? in the Resources section of this chapter.

How is the decision made as to which surgical procedure to use? Very little long-term scientific data exists for determining which procedure to choose for patients. The patient should be well informed about the differences among procedures and the options should center on the patient's history and individual risks versus benefits. Because no official systematic guidelines for each type of surgery exist, the choice of which surgery remains up to the patient, surgeon, and often to the available insurance and financial support.

Long-Term Success

The potential benefits of obesity and metabolic surgeries are strong motivating factors for patients who have been unsuccessful with other methods. Weight loss after bariatric surgery can be dramatic. The fastest weight loss occurs during the first 3 months, when dietary intake remains very restricted. After malabsorptive procedures, patients

BOX 8.3   Ineffective Surgical Treatments

Jaw Wiring

The concept of wiring the jaws together as a means to control weight was introduced in 1977. This orthodontic procedure, performed by dentists, prevented chewing and swallowing solid food, theoretically causing a reduction in calorie intake. Once the desired weight loss was achieved, the wiring was removed. Unfortunately the success rate of jaw wiring as a long-term method of achieving a normal weight was poor. Most patients did not learn to eat in a new, healthful manner. Some patients satisfied their hunger by sipping considerable amounts of high-calorie fluids through a straw so that they did not lose any weight at all. Large clinical studies demonstrated that a median weight loss of 55 lb was possible with jaw wiring but, after 4 months, the weight loss reached a plateau. When the wires were removed, patients regained 100% of the weight they had lost (Farquhar, 1986).

Liposuction

Liposuction is a popular form of cosmetic surgery that is intended to remove fat deposits under the skin from the abdomen, thighs, buttocks, neck, and back of arms. The fat is extracted with vacuum suction or with an ultrasonic probe that breaks up the fat and then removes it with suction. Though it seems as if this could be an effective way to lose excess fat, liposuction is not a cure for obesity. Relatively little body fat (less than 10 lb) can be removed safely and easily and the fat that is removed may come back with weight gain. In addition, deep visceral fat that is associated with metabolic derangements cannot be accessed easily with liposuction. While some physicians may have training before performing liposuction surgery, no standardized training is required and any licensed physician may perform the procedure. Because fat removal is considered a cosmetic procedure most medical insurance does not pay for liposuction (FDA, 2010).

can lose weight at the rate of 1 lb/day or as much as 90 lb in 3 months. This rapid rate of weight loss decreases by 6 to 9 months, and the peak in weight loss is achieved about 12 to 18 months after the procedure. Surgeons do not guarantee that individuals will reach an ideal body weight or a normal BMI range. The surgery commonly allows patients to reduce 50% of their excess body weight (EBW). Therefore, a person who weighs 300 lb and is 100 lb overweight could theoretically maintain a 50-lb loss. That individual would reach a long-term weight of about 250 lb and be healthier but still be in the overweight BMI category.

Even though surgical procedures produce large initial weight losses compared to diet, exercise, and medication, patients may not be more successful at maintaining weight loss when compared with individuals who have lost weight through nonsurgical means. A large intervention study in Sweden that assessed the effects of weight loss in severely obese patients showed that surgically treated subjects regained nearly a third of the weight that they lost by the 6-year follow-up (Karlsson, 2007). Research and clinical experience shows that weight regain after GBP occurs in approximately 20% of patients (Meguid, 2008). Weight regain after bariatric surgery occurs because anatomical and physiological adaptations that have occurred over time encourage a patient to return to those former eating and other lifestyle patterns that originally contributed to the development of obesity. Consuming high-calorie liquids or binge eating may allow for a progressive increase in total energy intake and weight regain. Surgery is not an easy fix for obesity because lifestyle and behavior modification are still needed to maintain successful long-term outcomes. In addition, success should be related to factors other than weight loss alone such as improvement of comorbidities, decreased mortality, enhanced quality of life, and positive psychosocial changes (Mechanick, 2008). Along with a comprehensive health team approach the surgeries may be seen as an additional tool that can help a person keep a commitment to following healthful eating and exercise patterns.

Insurance Coverage and Accessibility

Bariatric surgery costs an average of $17,000 to $26,000 and insurance coverage varies by state and insurance company. An individual's eligibility is subject to interpretation, and insurance denial of coverage is the most frequent reason for opting out of medically indicated weight-loss surgery (Kohn, 2009). A study of bariatric patients found that up to 30% of candidates do not receive bariatric surgery for reasons such as "unattainable prerequisites" (Al Harakeh, 2010). It was in an effort to improve insurers' acceptance of coverage of bariatric surgery procedures that the Centers of Excellence were identified by the ASMBS and the American College of Surgeons. In 2004, the United States Department of Health and Human Services reduced barriers to obtaining Medicare coverage for obesity treatments and now it endorses bariatric surgery as a safe and effective treatment for extreme obesity when performed at certified Centers of Excellence (USDHHS, 2004). The Medicare policy also removes a barrier to access in that it does not require potential patients to undergo dietary weight-loss plans ahead of time. The policies utilized by Medicare, the biggest insurer in the United States, are often followed by private insurers. While coverage for the surgery is offered by many insurance providers, postoperative care coverage remains limited in many instances. Because postoperative care remains an integral part of successful outcomes, patients and healthcare providers should advocate that insurance carriers cover follow-up care.

Future Techniques

Current bariatric surgery research is focused on the development of safer and less invasive techniques that hold promise for patient safety, recovery, and effectiveness (ASMBS, 2010). Many of the more prominent new technologies are incisionless and employ an endoscopic approach via a natural orifice such as the mouth. Two novel experimental procedures are the endoscopically delivered gastrointestinal liner and the gastric pacer. The gastric liner or endoluminal barrier is a nonsurgical way to bypass a portion the intestine (see **Figure 8.3**). It is a thin, flexible, tube-shaped liner that is placed endoscopically through the mouth and lines the first 2 ft of the small intestine. It forms a barrier between the food and the intestinal wall to prevent food from being absorbed while it passes through the liner. Placing this barrier is an outpatient procedure that does not require any surgery or incisions. It is intended to be temporary and can easily be removed. Theoretically, it should prevent absorption in the same areas of the gastrointestinal tract as a GBP procedure.

A gastric pacer is a device that consists of a pacemaker and a detector similar to a cardiac pacemaker. Two electrodes deliver an electrical impulse to the stomach or duodenal wall. When the patient eats or drinks, the pacemaker sends small electrical impulses that stimulate gastric nerves to send neurohumoral messages to the brain by means of nerves or the blood stream. Gastric pacemaker-produced impulses aim to artificially induce satiety so the individual experiences an early sensation of fullness. As a result, the person should feel less hungry, stop eating sooner than usual, and consume less food.

In 2003, researchers at the NIH formed a partnership with researchers called the Longitudinal Assessment of Bariatric Surgery, or LABS. The mission of LABS researchers is to plan and conduct studies that will lead to better understanding of bariatric surgery and its impact on the health and well-being of patients with extreme obesity (WIN, 2009). For more information on LABS, visit

FIGURE 8.3   Placement of endoluminal barrier.

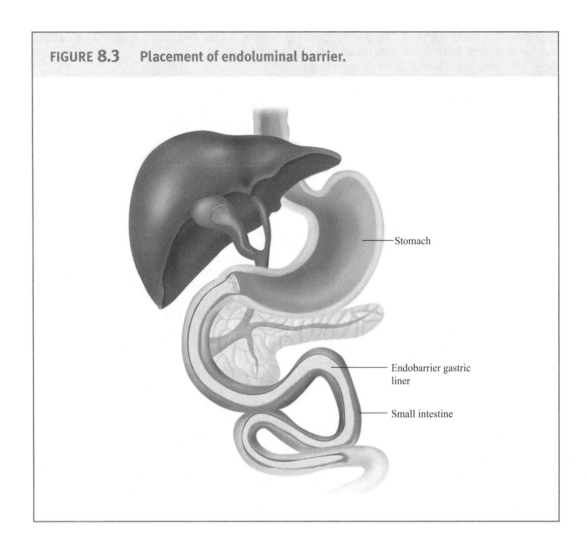

the LABS website listed in the Resources section of this chapter. Because of the large number of surgeries performed each year, basic research in the bariatric field has been enriched by data from clinical investigations and the availability of thousands of bariatric patients who can easily provide blood or tissue samples as part of the bariatric procedures. Studying data from these individuals can enhance scientific knowledge of the overall pathogenesis and pathophysiology of obesity. Directions for future basic research suggested at the 2004 ASBS Consensus Conference on Bariatric Surgery for Morbid Obesity include (Buchwald, 2005):

- Study interrelationships among specific bariatric surgical procedures, weight loss, variation in gastrointestinal hormones, and inflammatory markers.
- Explore the mechanisms by which different types of current bariatric procedures work

and how various bariatric surgical procedures regulate comorbid conditions of obesity.

- Gain insight into the basic causes and mechanisms of overweight and obesity.

Summary

Bariatric surgery is the most effective treatment for severe obesity in adults and adolescents. It produces significant weight loss, improvement of comorbid conditions, and longer life. While bariatric surgery is an appropriate treatment option for some, it is not a quick fix or a cure. It is the exchange of one set of medical issues for another. A commitment to lifestyle change is still necessary. Failure of the surgeries to produce adequate weight loss can occur if the reduced stomach pouch stretches, intestinal absorption increases, or diet and physical activity habits are not changed to support a lower body weight.

Two common procedures are gastric bypass (GBP) and laparoscopic adjustable gastric banding (LAGB). Both may be performed laparoscopically. Most experts view the GBP procedure as more durable, reliable, and effective because it encompasses both restrictive and malabsorptive aspects. It also brings about beneficial alterations in gastrointestinal hormones that regulate nutrient metabolism and satiety. Federal government agencies and private insurers have come to the opinion that GBP can be performed safely, particularly at high-volume Centers of Excellence. However, the technique remains challenging with potential serious complications (Nagle, 2010). LAGB is generally considered to be less invasive and safer than GBP, but the results may not be as effective for weight reduction in the long term. The choice of which specific operation is right for a particular patient should be individualized, and bariatric care should be supported both before and after surgery by multidisciplinary systems to ensure successful outcomes.

Because there is evidence that bariatric surgeries may be among the most effective treatments for metabolic conditions including type 2 diabetes, hypertension, and abnormal cholesterol levels, the procedures are now often referred to as metabolic and bariatric surgeries. This focus has led to new thinking that not only are the surgeries useful for weight loss, but they may also be appropriate for individuals with these metabolic derangements who are normal weight or only slightly overweight. As a caution against expanding bariatric surgery inappropriately, researcher Kenneth De Ville makes an argument that because bariatric surgery is an individual rather than population-based intervention and it is focused on *post facto* treatment rather than prevention, it should not be a primary response to the obesity health crisis (De Ville, 2010).

Critical Thinking Questions

Question: What should be the youngest eligible age for bariatric surgery? What factors are included in your decision?

Question: Considering a person your own age and sex, what specific changes in eating habits, lifestyle, and emotions would occur on a day-to-day basis after GBP or LAGB?

Question: What are the factors that contribute to weight regain even when the digestive tract is drastically altered with bariatric surgery?

Question: Measure out 1 or 2 oz, or about one-quarter cup, of some foods. How does the size of meals allowed after bariatric surgery compare with normal portions as described by USDA guidelines?

Resources

Longitudinal Assessment of Bariatric Surgery, or LABS
http://www.niddklabs.org

Teen-LABS
http://www.cincinnatichildrens.org/research/divisions/t/teen-labs/default/

AACE/TOS/ASMBS Guidelines
http://www.aace.com/pub/pdf/guidelines/Bariatric.pdf

https://www.aace.com/sites/default/files/Bariatric.pdf

AACE/TOS/ASMBS Guidelines, Table 9, Suggested Meal Progression after Roux-en-Y Gastric Bypass

AACE/TOS/ASMBS Guidelines, Table 10, Suggested Meal Progression after Laparoscopic Adjustable Gastric Band Procedure

Bariatric Surgery for Severe Obesity: What Are the Surgical Options? http://www.win.niddk.nih.gov/publications/gastric.htm

References

Adams TD, Gress RE, Smith SC, et al. Long-term mortality after gastric bypass surgery. *N Engl J Med*. 2007; 357:753–761.

Alami RS, Morton JM, Schuster R, et al. Is there a benefit to preoperative weight loss in gastric bypass patients? A prospective randomized trial. *Surg Obes Relat Dis*. Mar–Apr 2007;3(2):141–145; discussion 145–146.

Al Harakeh AB, Burkhamer KJ, Kallies KJ, Mathiason MA, Kothari SN. Natural history and metabolic consequences of morbid obesity for patients denied coverage for bariatric surgery. *Surg Obes Relat Dis*. Nov–Dec 2010;6(6):591–596.

ASMBS. Metabolic and Bariatric Surgery Fact Sheet. 2010;http://s3.amazonaws.com/publicASMBS/MediaPressKit/MetabolicBariatricSurgeryOverviewJuly2011.pdf. Accessed July 31, 2010.

Buchwald H. Bariatric surgery for morbid obesity: health implications for patients, health professionals, and third-party payers. *J Am Coll Surg*. Apr 2005;200(4): 593–604.

Buchwald H, Avidor Y, Braunwald E, et al. Bariatric surgery: a systematic review and meta-analysis. *JAMA*. Oct 13 2004;292(14):1724–1737.

Buchwald H, Estok R, Fahrbach K, et al. Weight and type 2 diabetes after bariatric surgery: systematic review and meta-analysis. *Am J Med*. Mar 2009;122(3): 248–256, e245.

Catona A, Gossenberg M, La Manna A, Mussini G. Laparoscopic gastric banding: preliminary series. *Obes Surg*. May 1993;3(2):207–209.

Christou NV, Sampalis JS, Liberman M, et al. Surgery decreases long-term mortality, morbidity, and health care use in morbidly obese patients. *Ann Surg*. Sep 2004;240(3):416–423; discussion 423–414.

Colles SL, Dixon JB, Marks P, Strauss BJ, O'Brien PE. Preoperative weight loss with a very-low-energy diet: quantitation of changes in liver and abdominal fat by serial imaging. *Am J Clin Nutr*. Aug 2006;84(2): 304–311.

De Ville K. Bariatric surgery, ethical obligation, and the life cycle of medical innovation. *Am J Bioeth*. Dec 2010;10(12):22–24.

Farquhar DL, Griffiths JM, Munro JF, Stevenson F. Unexpected weight regain following successful jaw wiring. *Scott Med J*. Jul 1986;31(3):180.

FDA. What Is Liposuction? 2010; http://www.fda.gov/MedicalDevices/ProductsandMedicalProcedures/SurgeryandLifeSupport/Liposuction/default.htm. Accessed August 15, 2010.

Jamal MK, DeMaria EJ, Johnson JM, et al. Insurance-mandated preoperative dietary counseling does not improve outcome and increases dropout rates in patients considering gastric bypass surgery for morbid obesity. *Surg Obes Relat Dis*. Mar–Apr 2006; 2(2):122–127.

Karlsson J, Taft C, Ryden A, Sjostrom L, Sullivan M. Ten-year trends in health-related quality of life after surgical and conventional treatment for severe obesity: the SOS intervention study. *Int J Obes (Lond)*. Aug 2007;31(8):1248–1261.

Kohn GP, Galanko JA, Overby DW, Farrell TM. Recent trends in bariatric surgery case volume in the United States. *Surgery*. Aug 2009;146(2):375–380.

Kremen AJ, Linner JH, Nelson CH. An experimental evaluation of the nutritional importance of proximal and distal small intestine. *Ann Surg*. Sep 1954;140(3): 439–448.

Kulick D, Hark L, Deen D. The bariatric surgery patient: a growing role for registered dietitians. *J Am Diet Assoc*. Apr 2010;110(4):593–599.

Lawson ML, Kirk S, Mitchell T, et al. One-year outcomes of Roux-en-Y gastric bypass for morbidly obese adolescents: a multicenter study from the Pediatric Bariatric Study Group. *J Pediatr Surg*. Jan 2006;41(1).

Livingston EH. The incidence of bariatric surgery has plateaued in the U.S. *Am J Surg*. Sep 2010a;200(3): 378–385.

Livingston EH. Surgical treatment of obesity in adolescence. *JAMA*. Feb 10 2010b;303(6):559–560.

Mechanick JI, Kushner RF, Sugerman HJ, et al. Executive summary of the recommendations of the American Association of Clinical Endocrinologists, the Obesity Society, and American Society for Metabolic & Bariatric Surgery medical guidelines for clinical practice for the perioperative nutritional, metabolic, and nonsurgical support of the bariatric surgery patient. *Endocr Pract*. Apr 2008;14(3): 318–336.

Meguid MM, Glade MJ, Middleton FA. Weight regain after Roux-en-Y: a significant 20% complication related to PYY. *Nutrition*. Sep 2008;24(9):832–842.

Nagle A. Bariatric surgery—a surgeon's perspective. *J Am Diet Assoc*. Apr 2010;110(4):520–523.

Nguyen NT, Paya M, Stevens CM, Mavandadi S, Zainabadi K, Wilson SE. The relationship between hospital volume and outcome in bariatric surgery at academic medical centers. *Ann Surg*. Oct 2004; 240(4):586–593; discussion 584–593.

NHLBI. National Heart, Lung, and Blood Institute. Clinical guidelines on the identification, evaluation, and treatment of overweight and obesity in adults: executive summary. Vol. No. 98-4083. Bethesda, MD: National Institutes of Health; 1998.

NIH. Gastrointestinal surgery for severe obesity. *Consensus Statement*. National Institutes of Health. Mar 25 1991;9:1–20.

Pories WJ, Dohm LG, Mansfield CJ. Beyond the BMI: the search for better guidelines for bariatric surgery. *Obesity (Silver Spring)*. May 2010;18(5):865–871.

Santry HP, Lauderdale DS, Cagney KA, Rathouz PJ, Alverdy JC, Chin MH. Predictors of patient selection in bariatric surgery. *Ann Surg*. Jan 2007;245(1):59–67.

Sjostrom L, Narbro K, Sjostrom CD, et al. Effects of bariatric surgery on mortality in Swedish obese subjects. *N Engl J Med*. Aug 23 2007;357(8):741–752.

Still CD, Benotti P, Wood GC, et al. Outcomes of preoperative weight loss in high-risk patients undergoing gastric bypass surgery. *Arch Surg*. Oct 2007;142(10): 994–998.

USDHHS. HHS Announces Revised Medicare Obesity Coverage Policy. U.S. Department of Health and Human Services News Release. 2004; http://archive.hhs .gov/news/press/2004pres/20040715.html.

WIN. Bariatric Surgery for Severe Obesity. Weight-control Information Network. 2009; http://www.win.niddk .nih.gov/publications/gastric.htm#normaldigest. Accessed July 31, 2010.

Woolford SJ, Clark SJ, Gebremariam A, Davis MM, Freed GL. To cut or not to cut: physicians' perspectives on referring adolescents for bariatric surgery. *Obes Surg*. Jul 2010;20(7):937–942.

Xanthakos SA. Bariatric surgery for extreme adolescent obesity: indications, outcomes, and physiologic effects on the gut-brain axis. *Pathophysiology*. Aug 2008;15(2):135–146.

CHAPTER 9

BEHAVIORAL ASPECTS OF WEIGHT MANAGEMENT

READER OBJECTIVES

- Summarize the reasons that behavior therapy learning theories are applicable to weight management
- Explain why it is necessary to assess readiness to lose weight and describe how the transtheoretical stages of change model may be applied to weight management
- Discuss how behavior therapy goal setting techniques may be used to develop realistic goals for weight management
- Describe the realistic expectations for long-term weight loss based on research studies about current interventions
- Name four behavioral strategies typically applied in behavior modification programs and review how the interaction of each of these strategies enhances behavior change success
- Assess the efficacy of group, individual, and technology-based behavior therapy programs for long-term weight management
- Compare and contrast the benefits and limitations of the Health at Every Size paradigm

CHAPTER OUTLINE

Behavior Therapy Assumptions and Characteristics

Living in an environment that encourages sedentary living and strongly promotes consumption of high-calorie foods requires conscious effort to overcome these barriers to good health. Along with dietary intervention, physical activity, pharmacotherapy, and bariatric surgery, behavioral modification is a vital aspect of obesity therapy (Levy, 2007). **Behavior therapy** is a specific form of psychotherapy. Behavior therapists do not focus on analyzing patient psychiatric disorders or searching for insight into the origins of their problem behaviors. For behavior therapists, the reasons behind behaviors are not as important as the fact that the behaviors can be changed. This therapeutic approach, also referred to as behavior modification therapy, is based on the underlying assumption that eating and physical activity patterns are learned behaviors and can be modified or replaced with more desirable actions (Wadden, 2007). The aim of behavior treatment for obesity is to help individuals develop skills to identify and modify their eating habits, activity level, and thinking and belief patterns that contribute to excess weight an obesity-related comorbidities (Foster, 2006).

Learned behaviors are often prompted by repeated antecedent events that become strongly linked with a particular response. Anyone who smells the aroma of baking cookies may be reminded about how good they taste or about a pleasant event where warm cookies were served. These thoughts can lead to a desire to eat even though the person is not at all hungry. With behavior therapy an individual learns to identify and discover ways to disconnect external factors (cookie aroma) and the internal factors (stimulated appetite) that trigger overeating so the effect of the trigger diminishes over time (Wadden, 2000). The following characteristics of behavioral therapy are effective for managing triggers (Wadden, 2000):

- Goal orientation: Goals are specified in clear and measurable terms.
- Process orientation: A set of learned behavioral skills are applied to weight management rather than relying on willpower.

- Small successive changes: Based on the learning principle of shaping, small incremental steps are used to achieve complex goals.

Behavior therapy for weight management is a continuing, multimodal process to assess readiness, establish goals, and apply behavior change techniques for individuals who may have varying degrees of motivation, expectations, skills, and support.

Assess Readiness to Lose Weight

An individual may understand the need to reduce weight or make lifestyle changes but not be ready to make a serious commitment. It is important for both dieters and healthcare professionals to assess readiness for weight loss, because in most cases anyone who is undecided or ambivalent about attempting weight management will not be successful. Healthcare providers may assume that patients will comply with weight-loss instructions without regard to patients' confidence or willingness. To optimize success for sustained weight management, a joint decision process between patients and providers is essential. Patients can share what they believe is possible for them to achieve based on their past experiences, and providers may use assessment techniques such as the transtheoretical, or stages of change, model to propose treatments and goals that are individualized and realistic for a patient at a given time.

Set Goals

Most overweight persons agree that to lose weight they need to eat less and exercise more, but figuring out how to accomplish these goals is not easy. Keeping goals specific and small and breaking down complex tasks into simple steps will increase the chance of success. Starting out with modest short-term goals allows for early success, which can increase motivation and the sense of self-efficacy. Using this technique involves detailed plans such as specific calorie goals and physical activity prescription, as well as keeping track with food and activity records.

BOX 9.1   Assessing Readiness with Stages of Change Model

As with other health behaviors, initiative for weight management may follow the transtheoretical stages of change model. The stages of change describe the sequence of behavioral and cognitive steps people use to make successful alterations in health behavior (Prochaska, 1994).

Applied to weight loss, the model describes the following stages:

1. Precontemplation—no intention to change or refusing to consider losing weight.
2. Contemplation—considering a weight-loss attempt.
3. Preparation—making a plan following the decision to lose weight.
4. Action—actively involved in weight control behaviors.
5. Maintenance—continuation of changed weight control behaviors after weight loss.
6. Relapse—reversion to adverse behavioral patterns and weight regain.

Individuals who indicate readiness (preparation or action stage) could benefit from targeted treatment. For those in the precontemplation or contemplation stage who are not yet ready to make a commitment, the immediate goal is to prevent further weight gain rather than a focus on weight loss. A person who has a relapse can be encouraged to determine why the lapse occurred and how a similar situation could be prevented in the future.

Data from: Prochaska JO, Velicer WF, Rossi JS, et al. Stages of change and decisional balance for 12 problem behaviors. *Health Psychol.* Jan 1994;13(1):39–46.

SMART Goals for Weight Management

To increase the likelihood of success and bring about a reinforcing sense of accomplishment, participants in behavior therapy are encouraged to set specific, quantifiable, realistic behavioral objectives that are time limited. A common behavioral tool is the SMART goals system. A website with a more complete description of this method of goal setting can be found in the Resources section in this chapter.

Although there is some variation in the terms used, the general SMART goal characteristics are:

S = Specific: Develop a specific goal instead of a more general one. The goal should be clear and unambiguous.

M = Measurable: A measurable goal allows assessment of progress toward successful outcome.

A = Attainable: Goals must be realistic and attainable. A goal is attainable if the goal-setter believes that it can be accomplished.

R = Relevant: A relevant goal represents an objective that is worthwhile and one that the goal-setter is willing and able to work toward. A relevant goal will encourage a desirable behavior that eventually becomes self-rewarding.

T = Timely: A commitment to a time frame or a target date helps to focus behavior change efforts.

Realistic Expectations

Even though scientific evidence suggests that a combination of a reduced-calorie diet, physical activity, and supportive behavioral modification methods are helpful, optimal objectives for weight loss or maintenance are not yet defined.

BOX 9.2 An Example of How a SMART Goal Is Set

An individual who is sedentary sets a goal of walking 20 minutes three times a week for the next month (Specific, Measurable, Timely). This person agrees that increasing physical activity is a worthwhile goal that can be reasonably accomplished (Relevant and Attainable). If this goal is attained, it may be renewed or another goal is set. If the goal is not reached a reevaluation is made and problem-solving skills can be applied to determine why the goal was not met.

NHLBI guidelines recommend weight loss of 1 to 2 lb/week and weight loss of 5 to 10% of body weight in obese patients as these aims have been shown to significantly reduce the risk and severity of weight-related comorbid conditions (NHLBI, 1998). This or any weight-loss plan should include discussion and agreement between patients or clients and providers as to the appropriate amount of weight loss and expectations about the time frame in which it should be achieved. To improve success for weight loss it is necessary to correct false beliefs and expectations as most individuals have unrealistic ideas about the magnitude of weight reduction that is possible with even the most intensive behavioral treatment.

Weight losses with most programs typically range from 7 to 10% of initial body weight, and the maximum amount of weight is lost during the first 6 months of treatment (Jeffery, 2000). Extremely obese patients, who have large amounts of excess weight to begin with, may lose a considerable amount of weight in absolute terms yet still remain obese or overweight. Unfortunately weight reduction is difficult to maintain as the mechanisms that cause weight regain such as hormonal feedback, decrease in metabolic rate, and/or a return to negative lifestyle habits are multifactorial. A major shortcoming of behavioral programs is the high likelihood that participants will regain weight once the treatment is ended. Without continued support individuals generally regain about one-third of weight loss within 1 year and nearly everyone experiences a complete regain within 5 years (Jeffery, 2000). Most participants in weight management programs are not satisfied with such modest results.

In a study reported in 2001, researchers asked nearly 400 women in a weight-loss program to describe their goal weight loss in terms of what they wished to achieve, what they would be happy with, and weight loss they would view as unsuccessful. The women hoped for an average of about a 38% reduction in body weight. A 25% reduction was described as "acceptable," but not one they would be happy with, and a 16% loss was considered "disappointing" (Foster, 1997). Although a weight reduction of 30% or more may be expected with bariatric surgery, it is more than three times the average weight loss that can be reasonably achieved with diet, exercise, and behavior therapy. This study suggests that unrealistic weight-loss goals are common among persons following a lifestyle modification plan. Even after a weight loss that significantly improves health or quality of life, they may feel unsuccessful.

In the case of physical activity, unrealistic expectations about the impact of exercise on weight loss may also need to be corrected. Addition of regular exercise to a low-calorie diet does not significantly increase weight loss as compared with diet alone (Wadden, 1997). Numerous studies have shown that once weight is lost high amounts of regular exercise (more than 300 minutes per week or about 40 to 45 minutes per day) are required to prevent regain (USDHHS, 2008).

As individuals discover that they are unable to meet their weight-loss goals, they might discount health benefits of their behavior changes and return to previous eating and activity habits and regain their lost weight as a result. Therefore, an important component of behavioral treatment is to prepare individuals to accept modest weight losses and to focus on realistic weight change that can be sustained over the long term. An alternative focus on nonweight outcomes such as improved metabolic measures or changes in quality of life such as increased energy, ability to play with children, or even how clothes fit may provide more immediate positive reinforcement.

Apply Behavior Modification Techniques

Behavioral therapy provides a wide variety of techniques that can be integrated into day-to-day decisions that eventually will be the basis of a healthful lifestyle. No single strategy has been shown to be superior, and using several components together appears to be associated with greater success (Wadden, 2000). Following are four behavioral strategies typically applied to weight loss and maintenance programs (Fujioka, 2002):

- Self-monitoring
- Stimulus control
- Cognitive restructuring
- Social support

Details and applications of these components have been described in self-help manuals such as the LEARN Program of Weight Management, and

their interrelationships are shown in **Figure 9.1** (Brownell, 2000).

Self-Monitoring

To change health behaviors, it helps for people to monitor and become aware of their actions such as overeating or being sedentary. Self-monitoring for weight management involves three major things; observing and recording all eating and exercise behaviors, and monitoring weight. Self-monitoring tools may include daily food diaries to record such items as types of foods consumed, total calorie intake, grams of fat or carbohydrate, or number of servings of fruit and vegetables. **Table 9.1** is an example of a daily food record and shows how to fill out a form for recording food amounts, eating times, and hunger levels. Records of physical activity may monitor exercise time, distance, or number of steps per day measured by a pedometer. For increased detail self-monitoring could also include information about times, places, and emotions associated with eating habits and activity levels. In addition, measures of percentage of body

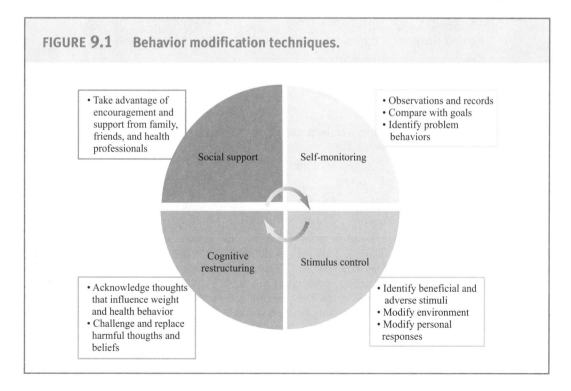

FIGURE 9.1   Behavior modification techniques.

TABLE 9.1   A Daily Food Record

Time	Amount	Food eaten	How prepared	How hungry am I? 0 = not hungry 5 = very hungry
6 am	1 cup	Nonfat milk		1
	2 cups	Bran flakes		
	2 Tbsp	Honey		
	2 cups	Black coffee	Brewed	
	2 Tbsp	Fat-free nondairy creamer	In coffee	
10 am	2 large (4-in. diameter)	Chocolate chip cookies	From grocery bakery	3
	1 16-oz bottle	Water		
Noon	2 slices	Turkey breast, deli sliced	In sandwich	4
	1 slice	American cheese	In sandwich	
	1 leaf	Leaf lettuce	In sandwich	
	2 slices	Tomato, sliced		
	1 Tbsp	Mustard	In sandwich	
	2 slices	Whole wheat bread	In sandwich	
	1 bag (1.4 oz)	Corn chips		
	12 oz	Diet root beer	Can	
5 pm	2 cups	Lasagna noodles with meat frozen dinner	Baked	4
	2 slices	Italian bread	Toasted	
	2 Tbsp	Olive oil mixed with garlic and herbs	Spread on toast	
8 pm	2 cups	Low-fat chocolate ice cream	In bowl	2

Example of how to keep track of foods eaten during the day

fat, waist circumference, blood pressure, or metabolic measures could be noted. The collected data can also be entered into a computerized analysis program such as the USDA MyPlate online interactive dietary and physical activity assessment tool (http://www.choosemyplate.gov). Results may be matched with personal goals set with the help of an Internet site such as MyPlate Intake Patterns.

The connection that can be made between self-monitoring observations and body weight or other health results is the cornerstone of behavioral treatment. It allows participants to appreciate how their lifestyle choices are helpful or harmful to their weight management efforts. A caveat about relying too strictly on self-monitoring data is that self-reporting on weight, diet, and activity records is not always very accurate. People generally underestimate how much they eat and overreport exercise (Kretsch, 1999). Even with nutrition education and training in the use of tools such as the

Nutrition Facts label on food packaging, estimating food and energy intake is difficult. Persons in the general population have been found to underestimate their calorie intake by 8 to 34% (de Vries, 1994). One study showed that overweight and obese individuals may have particularly inadequate self-monitoring skills, as their reports of calorie intake were underestimated and physical activity was overestimated by about 50% in each case (Lichtman, 1992).

Nonetheless, a journal with an accounting of all food and beverages consumed, physical activity, and weight changes is an effective learning tool since it provides immediate feedback. Problem patterns and cues become obvious, and possible solutions can be tried right away. Problem solving involves analyzing occurrences that might lead to inappropriate behavior such as overeating and then choosing new actions that are likely to improve success. Eating too fast? Reliance on fast foods? Finishing off the whole container of ice cream? Weight-control programs often suggest responses such as eating more slowly, having healthful foods on hand, planning ahead to avoid overly tempting eating situations, and basic education about realistic portion sizes and high- and low-calorie food choices.

The habit of frequently recording food intake has been shown to correlate with successful weight loss and individuals who regularly self-monitor their exercise are more likely to exercise and lose weight (Carels, 2005). Among 1,685 participants enrolled in a 20-week Dietary Approaches to Stop Hypertension (DASH) program, consistency with food diary recording was among the strongest predictors of weight change. Keeping a daily food diary was associated with an approximate 20 lb (44 kg) total weight loss compared with less than 10 lb (22 kg) lost by those who did not keep regular food diaries (Hollis, 2008). The importance of self-monitoring for weight loss was illustrated in a trial of a group of patients receiving both pharmaceutical therapy and lifestyle modification. Those who recorded their food intake regularly lost more than twice as much weight as those who recorded infrequently (18.1 versus 7.7 kg [40 versus 17 lb]) (Wadden, 2005). Furthermore, the National Weight Control Registry researchers report that self-monitoring is one of the techniques most frequently used among participants who have maintained weight loss (Wing, 2005).

Stimulus Control

In addition to monitoring food consumption and exercise, recording information about hunger levels, emotions, and social activities at the time of eating, can identify undesirable behaviors to be targeted for **stimulus control** techniques. Stimulus control is a key element used in behavioral therapy. This strategy is based on the presumption that much behavior is automatic and responsive to internal and external stimuli (Poston, 2000). According to the behavioral psychology principles of operant conditioning, reinforcing stimuli are those that increase the probability that a given action will be repeated. While it is impossible to control everything about the environment the overall idea is to eliminate signals for inappropriate eating and to increase the number of cues that foster healthy eating and exercise habits. Beneficial stimuli are those that reinforce healthful eating and exercise behaviors such as weight loss itself and improvements in health, body image, and quality of life (Fabricatore, 2007). Weight management guides, diet books, and websites provide extensive lists of tips and ideas for managing cues. Typical examples of practical stimulus control techniques include:

- Eat at the same time and place.
- Eat only at the table.
- Use smaller plates to make portions look bigger.
- Store tempting items out of sight.
- Have healthy snacks readily available.
- Avoid high-risk eating places such as fast food restaurants and all-you-can-eat buffets.
- Have walking shoes placed in a convenient spot where they will be a reminder.

To reduce adverse stimuli or undesirable factors that promote inactivity or eating in the absence of hunger, basic stimulus control methods focus on eliminating or modifying a response to those triggers (Poston, 2000). For example, if an individual eats when worried or stressed, preparing ahead to have appealing relaxation activities readily available provides positive alternative responses. Stimulus control also suggests that the act of eating should be a focus on its own. Turning off the television and refraining from reading during meals and snacks allows a state of mindfulness and the ability to concentrate on enjoying the eating experience.

Mindless Eating

Most people do not consistently eat too much just because they are hungry. Environmental and emotional triggers often override physiologic cues of satiation that direct when to stop eating. Tempting aromas or the appealing sight of food can stimulate unintended, or mindless, excess food consumption. Subconscious factors such as the amount, variety, and accessibility of food may also influence consumption of large portion sizes or increased frequency of eating (Wansink, 2004). To counteract these triggers, **mindfulness**, or a focus of attention and awareness on the present situation and circumstances, may make it easier to overcome habits and behaviors that result in overeating. Mindful eating is a concept that describes a nonjudgmental awareness of physical and emotional sensations associated with eating (Framson, 2009). More information about mindful eating and ways to structure surroundings to reduce the risk of mindless eating can be found in the Resources section of this chapter.

Stimulus Control Studies: Television Watching

On average, Americans spend more than 2.5 hours watching television each day (BLS, 2011). Research indicates that television-viewing time predicts waist circumference increases over a 5-year period in both men and women (Wijndaele, 2010). Television viewing may lead to weight gain through the mechanisms of increased sedentary behavior and food consumption (Hu, 2003). Another line of research suggests that dietary changes associated with television viewing may be the result of specific television content as much as total viewing time. A study that included both adults and children showed that participants consumed up to 45% more snack food when they were exposed to food commercials during television programming compared with watching the same program without the food commercials (Harris, 2009). The conclusions of studies such as these indicate that reducing total television viewing time may be a

useful tactic to create opportunities for increased physical activity and reduced caloric intake.

Cognitive Behavior Therapy

Education or instruction about a healthful lifestyle and skill in stimulus control tactics are necessary but generally are not sufficient to induce clinically significant weight loss. The dozens of daily decisions about food and activity behavior are also influenced by individual perceptions, thought patterns, and emotions such as anger, boredom, or even happiness that have nothing to do with hunger or external stimuli. A fundamental assumption of **cognitive behavioral therapy (CBT)** is that thoughts (or cognitions) have a direct influence on behaviors (Brownell, 2000). CBT emphasizes that it is imperative to acknowledge an individual's thought patterns when attempting behavior change. To this end, a CBT technique, cognitive restructuring, involves having clients become more aware of their self-perceptions and beliefs related to diet, body weight, and weight-loss expectations. Cognitive restructuring promotes self-efficacy, or an individual's belief that personal success is possible, by encouraging patients and clients to actively challenge and change negative internal dialogues to positive ones (Poston, 2000). Thoughts such as "I've had a stressful day, so I deserve to pass up my walk this evening and just relax" can be reframed or countered with thoughts more conducive to weight loss (for example, "I remember learning that exercise actually helps relieve stress—maybe I can take just 10 minutes to walk around the block"). A common cognitive distortion seen in weight-loss therapy is all-or-nothing thinking—particularly with regard to success or failure, unrealistic weight-loss goals, and exaggerated justifications for eating (for example, "I overate again; I am never going to have the willpower to lose weight so I may as well just finish off the cheesecake").

Behavioral therapy programs encourage participants to recognize these unrealistic standards, all-or-nothing thinking, and negative thoughts, and to replace them with more realistic and positive ideas. This focus on positive thoughts is a central feature of cognitive restructuring because it is common for obese patients to have poor self-esteem and body image (Poston, 2000). Obese patients who seek weight reduction may also suffer from significant depression or other psychological disturbance. These conditions may be associated with adverse food behaviors such as binge eating in which an individual eats a large amount of food in a short period of time and then feels out of control, ashamed, and distressed (Yanovski, 2003). For an overweight person with symptoms of depression, anxiety, or binge eating, typical CBT programs may not be adequate. These individuals may benefit from pharmacotherapy or treatment by a mental health professional before attempting to lose weight (Wadden, 2000).

Relapse Management

Lapses are a natural part of the weight-loss process and learning to anticipate and manage setbacks is an important aspect of behavioral treatment. Cognitive restructuring is useful in dealing with lapses or weight regain in that individuals are encouraged to see the setback for what it is: a temporary condition, from which it is possible to recover, instead of total failure. The setback is assessed to determine why the lapse occurred and how a similar situation could be prevented in the future. One technique is to acknowledge when loss of behavioral control is most likely. This may be at certain times, such as holidays, eating out, or at parties with friends. An appropriate response would be to rehearse ways to cope with those stimuli ahead of time. Each time a challenge is successfully managed the chances of relapse are reduced (Wadden, 2000).

Social Support Network

For relapse prevention or any aspect of weight management social support improves an individual's coping abilities when challenging situations arise. Social support may be gained from encouragement by a single individual or by reliance on a network of family, friends, workplace colleagues, and health professionals for confidence-building and emotional support. Research studies indicate individuals who perceive that they have more social support are more successful at weight loss and that having family members or spouses who

are supportive of weight management goals can be particularly helpful. In a meta-analysis of 12-month behavioral programs, mean weight loss was approximately 3 kg (6.6 lb) more in family-based interventions than in control programs where family members were not involved (Avenell, 2004).

Treatment Delivery Options

Behavioral therapy can be provided in either group or individual clinical settings, as commercial or peer-based weight-loss groups, or as self-help programs. Treatment sessions are typically conducted using a structured curriculum, such as the LEARN Program for Weight Management (Brownell, 2000) or the format used in the NIDDK Diabetes Prevention Program studies (Knowler, 2002). Sessions routinely focus on a review of participants' food and activity records and their progress toward personal goals. Lecturing from the group leader is minimized in favor of having participants ask questions or discuss their progress at each meeting. The primary objectives of meetings are to support success and to identify strategies to cope with problems or setbacks increasing the chance that eating and activity plans will continue to be followed. Homework that includes behavioral exercises and record keeping is a central component of lifestyle modification programs as maintaining diet and activity records is a consistent predictor of initial weight loss (Wadden, 2007).

Individual Versus Group Therapy

Most research indicates that either group or individual treatment settings may result in comparable long-term weight loss (Wadden, 2000). However, group sessions are popular because they provide more social support from others who are in the same challenging weight-control situations. Participants can take advantage of the lessons and successes of others in their peer group. Group treatment is also more cost-effective than individual care. Additionally, results of a study by Renjilian and colleagues (2001) suggested that one-on-one programs may be less effective than group programs. Weight loss was greater for participants who completed a 26-week behavior therapy program (11 kg [24.2 lb]) in the group format compared to those who received individual treatment (9.1 kg [20 lb]).

Internet-Based Programs

Time and travel demands associated with conventional face-to-face weight-loss programs may be a factor that contributes to an average program attrition rate of 20% in the first 6 months, with greater attrition occurring in longer courses (Polzien, 2007). Attending treatment sessions may be seen as a burden and many persons may prefer to lose weight without having to participate in structured programs (Manzoni, 2011). Therefore, developing alternative methods of delivering effective weight-loss programs that are appealing, accessible, and time- and cost-saving is a healthcare priority (Tate, 2001).

With the rapid increase in access to the Internet and the development of web-based commercial weight-loss programs several studies have begun to examine the effectiveness of behavioral treatments for weight loss or maintenance of weight loss achieved through online programs. A randomized trial reported that weight-loss maintenance over 18 months was comparable between participants in an Internet-based program and individuals who continued to meet in person (Harvey-Berino, 2004). In this study, it was attendance at meetings or chat room sessions, as well as frequency of self-monitoring that were highly related to successful maintenance. Wing and colleagues (2006) similarly found no significant differences in the maintenance of weight loss in more than 300 participants who attended either on-site or online maintenance sessions. These findings suggest that the Internet may be an effective medium to provide education and support for weight loss and weight-loss maintenance. The choice of an Internet-based or an in-person behavioral weight-loss program depends on whether a person prefers the convenience and possible lower cost of Internet programs or the face-to-face encouragement provided by individual or group sessions. An aspect of any successful program, whether online or in person, is that in addition to providing information it also provides some type of structure and frequent feedback or counseling.

In a 6-month trial overweight patients who were assigned to a structured Internet behavioral program lost more weight (4.1 kg [9 lb]) than those only given links to educational weight-loss websites (1.6 kg [3.5 lb]) (Tate, 2001). Another trial reported that adding behavioral counseling (e-counseling) to a general Internet weight-loss program resulted in greater weight reduction (4.4 kg [9.7 lb]) compared with subjects using the basic program only (2 kg [4.4 lb]) (Tate, 2003). It is particularly useful if participants can submit their food and activity records online and receive responses from a healthcare provider.

Long-Term Weight Maintenance

Consider what the health results would be if a short-term intervention of just a few weeks or months, with subsequent termination of medication, is applied in the case of diseases such as type 2 diabetes or hypertension. For both conditions, continuous, long-term management is necessary. Such a treatment plan would not be considered adequate or ethical. As is true of these and most chronic conditions, obesity also requires long-term therapy and management. Either with in-person or technology-based contact, improved long-term weight loss is enhanced by continued care after the initial phase of treatment. In a study of 80 obese women extended follow-up groups were compared with a no-contact group following a 20-week treatment program. The groups who were given extended contact maintained a significantly greater percentage of their initial weight loss 12 months after treatment. A larger percentage of follow-up participants achieved losses of 10% or more in body weight compared with the no-contact participants (35% versus 6%) (Perri, 2001). Studies by Wadden (1994) and Wing (1994) also showed weight-loss maintenance was prolonged during the time subjects attended follow-up sessions.

Ongoing contact provides the support and motivation that is needed to continue to practice weight-control skills. One might assume from these results that if treatment could continue indefinitely, maintenance of any goal weight could be achieved. However, over time a decline in participant interest or ability to continue to take part in weight-loss programs occurs. Unfortunately success at weight management generally declines over time even with the best programs. The concerted effort required to persevere with a restrictive diet and a large amount of physical activity over a long time period is difficult to sustain. The reinforcing properties of food consumption may be more robust or appealing than those associated with maintaining a lower body weight. While long-term behavioral treatment clearly improves the maintenance of weight loss, extending the length of treatment is effective for delaying—not preventing—weight regain (Jeffrey, 2000).

Health at Every Size

Because weight regain is the most frequent long-term outcome of exercise, dietary restriction, and behavior modification treatment, there is an imperative need for alternative approaches to achieving good health. An innovative weight paradigm with the trademarked name **Health at Every Size®** (HAES) shifts the emphasis from the traditional weight-centered treatments to a focus on size acceptance and achieving a healthy lifestyle without dieting. Dieting may have unintended consequences such as contributing to repeated cycles of weight loss and regain, eating disorders, distraction from other personal health goals, reduced self-esteem, and stigmatization and discrimination. The HAES program is not based on weight loss but on supporting overall health for everyone (Bacon, 2011). HAES encourages size acceptance and heightened awareness and response to body signals and it discourages weight and size prejudice. The HAES philosophy rejects the view that the numbers on a scale, or that height/weight charts can determine an appropriate weight for an individual or BMI categories apply to everyone. Instead, the conceptual framework of this approach is based on issues such as (Robson, 2005):

- Acceptance of the natural diversity in body shape and size. It encourages an affirmation of human beauty and worth regardless of weight, physical size, and shape.

- Awareness about ineffectiveness of dieting for weight loss.
- Use of internal cues such as hunger and fullness rather than external cues such as calories to guide eating behavior.
- Enhanced knowledge about the physiological and environmental bases of body weight.
- Improved self-esteem and body image through self-acceptance rather than weight loss.
- Health benefits of physical activity for enjoyment and enhanced quality of life.

The HAES practice does not suggest that removing emphasis on body weight implies that it is acceptable to ignore health risks and medical problems. HAES advocates that the treatments for medical conditions be applied similarly to thin and overweight persons. In the case of hypertension, for example, standards of care suggest that dietary changes, increases in physical activity, stress management, and medication, if necessary, can be used to successfully manage the disease. All those therapies should be offered regardless of BMI. Patients with type 2 diabetes are sometimes threatened with having to take insulin shots if they do not lose weight. The primary purpose of diabetes treatment is not to alter body weight but to normalize blood glucose as efficiently and effectively as possible. Adopting the HAES approach may help healthcare professionals, dietitians, nurses, and physicians, to be nonjudgmental of their patients with obesity and to treat comorbidities rather than have their patients agree to or attempt to reduce weight first.

Research about HAES has shown inconsistent results that are generally comparable in effectiveness to diet, exercise, and behavioral treatments. Reports from weight-acceptance intervention studies found that, while significant weight loss usually does not occur, there could be beneficial effects on certain eating behaviors. A study conducted at the University of California, Davis, where HAES was compared with an energy-restricted diet, showed that after 1 year, the diet group lost an average of 5.9 kg (13 lb) whereas the HAES group weight did not change significantly (Bacon, 2002). However, the obese female chronic dieters who participated in the HAES program were more likely to maintain long-term favorable behavior changes and health improvements as compared to a control group that participated in the traditional diet program. It should be noted that the HAES group did have a more intensive intervention (Bacon, 2005). Researchers at Laval University in Canada compared eating behaviors of women who participated in either a HAES group, a social support group, or a control group. It was found that food intake in response to perception of hunger was significantly lower at a 1-year follow-up in both the HAES and social support groups when compared to the control group. In addition, disinhibition, or overeating in response to impulses or situational lack of control of food intake, was significantly lower in the HAES group than in the control group. While the HAES approach did seem to have improvements on eating behaviors related to disinhibition and hunger, the outcomes were not different from those in the social support intervention (Provencher, 2009).

Advocates of HAES emphasize that the approach encourages individualized exercise habits, and they point to scientific evidence that shows benefits of physical activity on cardiorespiratory fitness and reduced chronic disease even without any weight loss. Reports have shown that obese individuals who are active and fit have lower mortality rates than normal-weight persons who are inactive and unfit (Church, 2004). Owing to psychological health benefits that include improved self-esteem, the fat acceptance movement promotes HAES. The National Association to Advance Fat Acceptance (NAAFA) is an organization whose members are primarily overweight and obese women who have repeatedly tried dieting to control their weight but have not succeeded. It also promotes overall physical and emotional health for members without regard to body size.

There are challengers to the concept of HAES. Philosophical arguments against it are best summarized by the argument made by Deidre Barrett, a psychologist at Harvard University. She approaches obesity from an evolutionary standpoint and asserts, "Our instincts are designed for the African savannah, not food courts" (Barrett, 2007). She comments that if we follow our instincts to forage, which are made easier by vending machines, obesity is the predictable result. Barrett further argues that overweight individuals and populations need to make radical behavior changes that are biologically easier than making gradual changes in lifestyle.

Bariatric surgeons, whose patients are very obese, may also have a difference of opinion about the value of HAES. Bariatric surgery usually results in rapid, large changes in body weight that can have an immediate impact on metabolic dysfunction, and, for people who are severely obese, bariatric surgery is an obvious option to decrease diseases associated with obesity. For some obese individuals, interventions not directly aimed at weight loss can enhance psychological well-being, and it could be advantageous to use both HAES and bariatric surgery together (Tanco, 1998). More information about HAES and the researchers and supporters who advocate its use can be seen on websites that are listed in the Resources section of this chapter. The nondieting approach represents an interesting development in the care of obese persons. However, efficacy claims need to be tested by more studies that measure metabolic and cardiovascular risk factors associated with nondieting interventions. Those results will allow individuals to make informed decisions about managing their physical and emotional health.

Summary

Lifestyle modification, which involves applying behavior therapy principles to bring about changes in diet and physical activity patterns, is the foundation of obesity treatment. Even when pharmacotherapy or bariatric surgeries are used people with obesity must make significant lifestyle alterations in order to experience long-term success. Because individuals interested in weight management have varying degrees of motivation, expectations, skills, and support, behavior therapy includes the processes of assessing readiness, establishing goals, and applying a variety of behavior change techniques to individualize treatment. To optimize the possibility of sustained weight management, goal setting should be a joint decision process with agreement between patients and providers. Because most people have mistaken ideas about how quickly and how much weight can be lost, an important component of behavioral treatment is to shift the focus to realistic modest weight losses that can be sustained over the long term.

Most of the lifestyle modification programs have several behavioral techniques in common including self-monitoring, stimulus control, cognitive restructuring, and social support. Behavioral therapy treatment sessions use a structured curriculum and provide intensive and frequent feedback and counseling to support participants' attempts at lifestyle changes.

The meetings may be in a group or an individual clinical setting or even provided through web-based programs. Group sessions are popular because they provide social support; however, for some, attending treatment sessions may be seen as a burden and the attrition rate is 20% or more. A major limitation of all behavioral programs is the high probability that participants will regain weight.

Participants in behavioral therapy programs maintain on average about two-thirds of their initial weight loss 12 months after treatment termination. In studies with extended follow-up, clients return gradually to baseline within about 5 years. An alternative focus on nonweight outcomes such as improved metabolic measures or changes in quality of life may provide more acceptable and satisfying end points. Health At Every Size (HAES) is an innovative concept that shifts the emphasis from traditional weight-centered interventions to a focus on size acceptance and a healthy lifestyle without dieting.

A continuous-care model of lifestyle intervention that views obesity as a chronic disease requiring support or contact after the conclusion of formal treatment increases long-term maintenance and delays regain. It is clear that treatment of obesity once it has occurred is not the answer to combating the obesity epidemic. A more constructive response might be to implement behavioral principles and dietary and physical activity interventions as public health policy in homes, schools, and workplaces.

Critical Thinking Questions

Question: What reasons may individuals give for not being ready to lose weight?

Question: What would help them move to a precontemplation or contemplation stage?

Question: What types of activities would you expect from a person who is in the preparation stage for weight loss?

Question: What ideas can you provide to help extend the maintenance phase and to prevent relapse?

Question: If you had an obesity clinic what behavioral therapy options would you include in your weight management program? Why have you chosen these options? Who would be the best people to provide these interventions?

Question: From your experience with educational and interactive sites on the Internet, do you think this technology can be useful for weight management? Which aspects of web-based programs would be most beneficial and which would have a negative effect?

Question: What is your opinion about programs that take the focus off of weight loss and direct efforts to improving relationship with food, physical activity, and body image? Could that be helpful in decreasing health risks associated with obesity?

Resources

Goal Setting with the SMART Technique
http://www.smartgoalsacronym.com/
The Center for Mindful Eating
http://www.tcme.org/
This site has more information on how and why to practice mindfulness.
Brian Wansink's Mindless Eating Website
http://mindlesseating.org/
This site has ideas about structuring surroundings and tools and links to reduce the risk of mindless eating.
Health at Every Size
http://www.cdc.gov/chronicdisease/resources/publications/aag/obesity.htm
http://www.naafa.org
http://www.lindabacon.org/
http://jonrobison.net/

References

Avenell A, Broom J, Brown TJ, et al. Systematic review of the long-term effects and economic consequences of treatments for obesity and implications for health improvement. *Health Technol Assess*. May 2004;8(21):iii–iv, 1–182.

Bacon L, Aphramor L. Weight science: evaluating the evidence for a paradigm shift. *Nutr J.* 2011;10:9.

Bacon L, Keim NL, Van Loan MD, et al. Evaluating a 'non-diet' wellness intervention for improvement of metabolic fitness, psychological well-being and eating and activity behaviors. *Int J Obes Relat Metab Disord.* Jun 2002;26(6):854–865.

Bacon L, Stern JS, Van Loan MD, Keim NL. Size acceptance and intuitive eating improve health for obese, female chronic dieters. *J Am Diet Assoc.* Jun 2005; 105(6):929–936.

Barrett D. Waistland: The Revolutionary Science Behind Our Weight and Fitness Crisis. New York: W.W. Norton & Co.; 2007.

BLS. Bureau of Labor Statistics. American Time Use Survey—2009 Results. 2010; http://www.bls.gov/news.release/pdf/atus.pdf. Accessed July 10, 2010.

Brownell KD, LEARN Education Center. *The LEARN Program for Weight Management 2000: Lifestyle, Exercise, Attitudes, Relationships, Nutrition.* Dallas: American Health; 2000.

Carels RA, Darby LA, Rydin S, Douglass OM, Cacciapaglia HM, O'Brien WH. The relationship between self-monitoring, outcome expectancies, difficulties with eating and exercise, and physical activity and weight loss treatment outcomes. *Ann Behav Med.* Dec 2005;30(3):182–190.

Church TS, Cheng YJ, Earnest CP, et al. Exercise capacity and body composition as predictors of mortality among men with diabetes. *Diabetes Care.* Jan 2004; 27(1):83–88.

de Vries JH, Zock PL, Mensink RP, Katan MB. Underestimation of energy intake by 3-d records compared with energy intake to maintain body weight in 269 nonobese adults. *Am J Clin Nutr.* Dec 1994;60(6): 855–860.

Fabricatore AN. Behavior therapy and cognitive-behavioral therapy of obesity: is there a difference? *J Am Diet Assoc.* Jan 2007;107(1):92–99.

Foster G. The behavioral approach to treating obesity. *Am Heart J.* Mar 2006;151(3):625–627.

Foster GD, Wadden TA, Vogt RA, Brewer G. What is a reasonable weight loss? Patients' expectations and evaluations of obesity treatment outcomes. *J Consult Clin Psychol.* Feb 1997;65(1):79–85.

Framson C, Kristal AR, Schenk JM, Littman AJ, Zeliadt S, Benitez D. Development and validation of the mindful eating questionnaire. *J Am Diet Assoc.* Aug 2009;109(8):1439–1444.

Fujioka K. Management of obesity as a chronic disease: nonpharmacologic, pharmacologic, and surgical options. *Obes Res.* Dec 2002;10 Suppl 2:116S–123S.

Harris JL, Bargh JA, Brownell KD. Priming effects of television food advertising on eating behavior. *Health Psychol.* Jul 2009;28(4):404–413.

Harvey-Berino J, Pintauro S, Buzzell P, Gold EC. Effect of internet support on the long-term maintenance of weight loss. *Obes Res.* Feb 2004;12(2):320–329.

Hollis JF, Gullion CM, Stevens VJ, et al. Weight loss during the intensive intervention phase of the weight-loss maintenance trial. *Am J Prev Med.* Aug 2008; 35(2):118–126.

Hu FB, Li TY, Colditz GA, Willett WC, Manson JE. Television watching and other sedentary behaviors in relation to risk of obesity and type 2 diabetes mellitus in women. *JAMA.* Apr 9 2003;289(14):1785–1791.

Jeffery RW, Drewnowski A, Epstein LH, et al. Long-term maintenance of weight loss: current status. *Health Psychol.* Jan 2000;19(1 Suppl):5–16.

Knowler WC, Barrett-Connor E, Fowler SE, et al. Reduction in the incidence of type 2 diabetes with lifestyle intervention or metformin. *N Engl J Med.* Feb 7 2002;346(6):393–403.

Kretsch MJ, Fong AK, Green MW. Behavioral and body size correlates of energy intake underreporting by obese and normal-weight women. *J Am Diet Assoc.* Mar 1999;99(3):300–306; quiz 307–308.

Levy RL, Finch EA, Crowell MD, Talley NJ, Jeffery RW. Behavioral intervention for the treatment of obesity: strategies and effectiveness data. *Am J Gastroenterol.* Oct 2007;102(10):2314–2321.

Lichtman SW, Pisarska K, Berman ER, et al. Discrepancy between self-reported and actual caloric intake and exercise in obese subjects. *N Engl J Med.* Dec 31 1992;327(27):1893–1898.

Manzoni GM, Pagnini F, Corti S, Molinari E, Castelnuovo G. Internet-based behavioral interventions for obesity: an updated systematic review. *Clin Pract Epidemiol Ment Health.* 2011;7:19–28.

NHLBI. National Heart, Lung, and Blood Institute. Clinical guidelines on the identification, evaluation, and treatment of overweight and obesity in adults: executive summary. Vol. No. 98-4083. Bethesda, MD: National Institutes of Health; 1998.

Perri MG, Nezu AM, McKelvey WF, Shermer RL, Renjilian DA, Viegener BJ. Relapse prevention training and problem-solving therapy in the long-term management of obesity. *J Consult Clin Psychol.* Aug 2001; 69(4):722–726.

Polzien KM, Jakicic JM, Tate DF, Otto AD. The efficacy of a technology-based system in a short-term behavioral weight loss intervention. *Obesity (Silver Spring).* Apr 2007;15(4):825–830.

Poston WS, Hyder ML, O'Byrne KK, Foreyt JP. Where do diets, exercise, and behavior modification fit in the treatment of obesity? *Endocrine.* Oct 2000;13(2): 187–192.

Prochaska JO, Velicer WF, Rossi JS, et al. Stages of change and decisional balance for 12 problem behaviors. *Health Psychol.* Jan 1994;13(1):39–46.

Provencher V, Begin C, Tremblay A, et al. Health-At-Every-Size and eating behaviors: 1-year follow-up results of a size acceptance intervention. *J Am Diet Assoc.* Nov 2009;109(11):1854–1861.

Renjilian DA, Perri MG, Nezu AM, McKelvey WF, Shermer RL, Anton SD. Individual versus group therapy for obesity: effects of matching participants to their treatment preferences. *J Consult Clin Psychol.* Aug 2001;69(4):717–721.

Robison J. Health at every size: toward a new paradigm of weight and health. *MedGenMed.* 2005;7(3):13.

Tanco S, Linden W, Earle T. Well-being and morbid obesity in women: a controlled therapy evaluation. *Int J Eat Disord.* Apr 1998;23(3):325–339.

Tate DF, Jackvony EH, Wing RR. Effects of Internet behavioral counseling on weight loss in adults at risk for type 2 diabetes: a randomized trial. *JAMA.* Apr 9 2003;289(14):1833–1836.

Tate DF, Wing RR, Winett RA. Using Internet technology to deliver a behavioral weight loss program. *JAMA.* Mar 7 2001;285(9):1172–1177.

USDHHS. Physical Activity Guidelines Advisory Committee Report. 2008; http://www.health.gov/paguidelines/. Accessed March 3, 2010.

Wadden TA, Berkowitz RI, Womble LG, et al. Randomized trial of lifestyle modification and pharmacotherapy for obesity. *N Engl J Med.* Nov 17 2005;353(20): 2111–2120.

Wadden TA, Butryn ML, Wilson C. Lifestyle modification for the management of obesity. *Gastroenterology.* May 2007;132(6):2226–2238.

Wadden TA, Foster GD. Behavioral treatment of obesity. *Med Clin North Am.* Mar 2000;84(2):441–461, vii.

Wadden TA, Foster GD, Letizia KA. One-year behavioral treatment of obesity: comparison of moderate and severe caloric restriction and the effects of weight maintenance therapy. *J Consult Clin Psychol.* Feb 1994;62(1):165–171.

Wadden TA, Vogt RA, Andersen RE, et al. Exercise in the treatment of obesity: effects of four interventions on body composition, resting energy expenditure, appetite, and mood. *J Consult Clin Psychol.* Apr 1997;65(2):269–277.

Wansink B. Environmental factors that increase the food intake and consumption volume of unknowing consumers. *Annu Rev Nutr.* 2004;24:455–479.

Wijndaele K, Healy GN, Dunstan DW, et al. Increased cardiometabolic risk is associated with increased TV viewing time. *Med Sci Sports Exerc.* Aug 2010; 42(8):1511–1518.

Wing RR, Blair E, Marcus M, Epstein LH, Harvey J. Year-long weight loss treatment for obese patients with type II diabetes: does including an intermittent very-low-calorie diet improve outcome? *Am J Med.* Oct 1994;97(4):354–362.

Wing RR, Phelan S. Long-term weight loss maintenance. *Am J Clin Nutr.* Jul 2005;82(1 Suppl):222S–225S.

Wing RR, Tate DF, Gorin AA, Raynor HA, Fava JL. A self-regulation program for maintenance of weight loss. *N Engl J Med.* Oct 12 2006;355(15): 1563–1571.

Yanovski SZ. Binge eating disorder and obesity in 2003: could treating an eating disorder have a positive effect on the obesity epidemic? *Int J Eat Disord.* 2003;34 Suppl:S117–S120.

CHAPTER 10

WHERE DOES RESPONSIBILITY LIE?

READER OBJECTIVES

- Discuss the roles of families and schools in preventing childhood obesity
- Summarize possible adverse and beneficial effects of the built environment on obesity
- Explain why many worksites promote obesity
- Describe and assess proposed and existing responses to the obesity epidemic from each of these stakeholders:
  - Healthcare providers
  - Schools
  - Worksites
  - Public health
  - State and community government and organizations
  - National Programs
  - Industry
- Interpret the implications of obesity-related food and beverage taxes and liability legislation
- Describe how several national programs put into place after 2008 may help reduce obesity in America

CHAPTER OUTLINE

Where Does Responsibility Lie?

Who is at fault for the high prevalence of obesity? Is it that individuals have become lazy and irresponsible with their food choices? Are fast food chains and advertisers the cause? Can genetic predisposition to store excess fat be blamed? Studies have shown that it is a combination of personal food choices, lack of exercise, environmental circumstances, and genetic disposition that all play a role. Obesity is becoming recognized as a problem that encompasses both personal and collective responsibility. In a 2009 national poll adults were asked about reasons for the increasing rate of obesity in America. An adverse food environment was the highest-ranking cause while the lowest-rated was irresponsible behavior such as sloth and gluttony. In addition, the group acknowledged that there are multiple reasons that obesity occurs including time crunch issues, addiction to certain foods, and pressures from food marketers. The participants in this study supported government interventions to improve school nutrition (69%) and even a ban on junk-food advertising (51%) (Barry, 2009). As one in three Americans are obese, there is increasing public awareness that this is a health issue for which individuals, families, healthcare providers, schools, government, and the business community must be willing to invest time, energy, and resources to solve.

Individuals

In the past, approaches to obesity treatment have largely focused on individual behaviors as the cause of obesity. This view is consistent with the American values of individualism, self-determination, and morality in which people are responsible for their personal situation (Brownell, 2010). Hard work, determination, and self-discipline create success (e.g., weight loss) and failure reflects personal weakness and self-indulgence (Puhl, 2009). Many people overeat even when they want to lose weight. Eating brings immediate gratification whereas possible benefits of food restriction or control occur only in the future. Professionals' attitudes toward weight control fluctuate between empowering individuals to manage their weight and blaming them when they fail to do so. Based on the notion that Americans must lack sufficient knowledge of those

behaviors that lead to weight gain, education has been the most common intervention.

Approaches at all levels are geared to providing information and to motivating individuals to make informed choices and modify their behaviors. This focus comes from healthcare providers, obesity books and websites, and even the federal government. In 2004, the United States Department of Health and Human Services (USDHHS) launched the "Small Steps" campaign, funded at $1.5 million annually, to increase awareness about overweight and obesity (Puhl, 2010). This, or any type of government intervention that aims to improve an individual's health, is perceived by some as promotion of a "nanny" state and an intrusion on personal freedoms. However, there are arguments that the environment profoundly affects the scope of everyone's food choices. For example, children at home or in a school cafeteria may select what they put on their plates, but which choices they make is influenced by the availability of some foods and not others (Brownell, 2010).

Families

For both adults and children healthful eating habits and physical activity should be a family affair. Obesity prevention is best initiated during childhood. Adults are commonly the food policymakers at home because young children usually do not do the grocery shopping or food preparation themselves. Studies demonstrate that children's health behavior is strongly influenced by parent role modeling. When children see adults eating a variety of nutritious foods and valuing physical activity they will be more likely to accept those habits (Scaglioni, 2008). Parents are cautioned not to let their children get fat, and they are held responsible for feeding their children properly. Providing healthful foods for children can be a challenge because the definition of "healthy food" has been evolving. According to the FDA's 2010 Dietary Guidelines for Americans, the major part of a healthy diet consists of whole foods such as fresh fruits, vegetables, whole grains, low-fat dairy, and lean meats. While candy, chips, and sodas are not included parents are often persuaded to show their children how much they love them by rewarding them with these highly advertised treats.

An article in the *Journal of the American Medical Association* (*JAMA*) raised some controversial issues. Should parents of extremely obese children face legal action? Can obesity in young children be a sign of parental abuse? The authors suggested that severe obesity (child BMI above the 99th percentile) "represents profoundly dysfunctional eating and exercising habits" that lead to health problems indicative of child abuse and neglect (Murtagh, 2011). A news article about a couple from Georgia shows a dramatic application of the issue. They were arrested and charged with felony child cruelty of their 5-year-old daughter who lived in filthy conditions, weighed 158 pounds, and could barely walk a few feet. The child was taken into protective custody (Malone, 2011). According to the Centers for Disease Control (CDC), the average 5-year-old girl weighs around 50 pounds (CDC, 2010). In another case, the mother of a 555-pound 14-year-old boy from South Carolina was arrested and charged with criminal neglect. The boy was put in foster care (Barnett, 2009). The authors of the *JAMA* paper write that protective custody may serve a child's best interests and may be the only realistic way to control life-threatening obesity of children like these. The study's coauthor, David Ludwig, says removing children from such homes "ideally will support not just the child but the whole family, with the goal of reuniting child and family as soon as possible" (Murtagh, 2011).

Parents have a constitutional right to raise their children as they choose, though the state may intervene to protect children from abuse. Federal law defines child abuse and neglect as "any recent act or failure to act on the part of a parent or caretaker, which results in death, serious physical or emotional harm … or an act or failure to act which presents an imminent risk of serious harm" (Dodd, 2010). Undernourishment and failure to thrive caused by inadequate feeding practices are conditions that have previously been the focus of child abuse and neglect laws. As the number of severely obese children increases, it is conceivable that these same laws will be applied more often to childhood obesity.

Environment: Food and Physical Activity Accessibility

An individual's eating and physical activity behaviors do not occur in a vacuum. Social and economic influences have altered the environment to one that promotes and reinforces obesity. Humans are highly responsive to environmental cues such as availability, pricing, and marketing. These powerful forces make it difficult to make responsible choices (Brownell, 2010). In the context of individual and public health the environment is defined as the sum of influences from all surroundings, opportunities, or conditions of life. Health researchers have found that the **built environment**, or those human-generated aspects of a living space, can significantly affect weight status (Papas, 2007). **Table 10.1** shows examples of various dimensions of the built environment.

A person who lives close to shopping, schools, public transportation, or a park will probably get more exercise than a person living where there is a lack of sidewalks or community playgrounds and where being outside may not be safe. In addition someone who lives in an area with few supermarkets and a fast food outlet on nearly every block is likely to eat more fast food than an individual who lives where fresh produce and nutritious food is easily accessible. Educational efforts to provide nutritional guidance or to change dietary habits will be ineffective if it is too difficult or too expensive for people to get to stores that carry healthier foods. About 23 million Americans live in cities and rural districts, especially in lower-income areas, where there is no easy access to an affordable, full-service supermarket that offers fresh fruits and vegetables. Such places are known as **food deserts** (Treuhaft, 2010). Residents of these neighborhoods typically rely on fast food restaurants, convenience stores, or smaller neighborhood stores that may not carry healthy foods or may offer them only at higher prices (Ver Ploeg, 2009).

Schools

Young people spend more time at school than any other place except their homes. More than 90% of students eat lunch in school, and about 20% also eat breakfast there. Food at school can make up as much as 40% of a student's daily energy intake (Briefel, 2009). Unfortunately many schools provide a predominance of high-fat, high-sugar foods and beverages in cafeterias, school stores, and vending machines. On the energy expenditure side, fewer children walk or bicycle to school

TABLE 10.1   Dimensions of the Built Environment

Definition of built environment	Dimensions	Examples
It encompasses all buildings, spaces, and products that are created, or modified, by people.	Food choices Physical activity choices Support for good health Safety	Grocery store choices Fast food outlets Workplace vending machine choices Famers' markets Opportunity for gardening Walking/biking pathways Parks and playgrounds Public transportation Every part of the environment that affects physical activity in daily routines and lifestyles
It includes homes, schools, workplaces, parks, recreation areas, business areas, and transportation systems.		
It includes land-use planning and policies that impact communities in urban, rural, and suburban areas.		

(McDonald, 2007), and there is reduced time for physical education, recess, and other physical activity in response to budget concerns and pressures to improve academic test scores.

Worksites

Innovation, automation, and labor-saving devices have resulted in fewer workers in primary industries such as agriculture, fishing, mining, or forestry, and large increases in the proportion of people whose worksites are not designed to encourage movement. A study of shifts in the labor force since 1960 shows that jobs requiring moderate physical activity, which accounted for 50% of the labor market in 1960, declined to just 20% by 2008. The shift translates to an average reduction of about 120 to 140 calories a day that had been required for on-the-job physical activity. The authors suspect that these unused calories are a significant contributor to the steady weight gain in the United States over the past five decades (Church, 2011). The majority of workplaces require low energy expenditure, and they are also places where access to energy-dense food and beverages is common. Snacks, candy, and pastries are often used to reward and motivate employees. It can be challenging to turn down doughnuts brought in by the boss or homemade desserts from a coworker.

Epidemiologic studies of characteristics of working conditions and worker overweight or obesity have shown associations between greater BMI and long work hours, shift work, and job stress (Schulte, 2007).

Advertising

The food industry spends billions of dollars each year to develop products, packaging, and marketing techniques that entice consumers to buy their products. Marketers place commercials on television, the Internet, radio, video games, toys, movies, and billboards to reach their target audiences. Impressionable young children are particularly easy targets for the food industry. Studies show that children as young as 2 years demonstrate a preference for foods they see on television commercials versus nonadvertised foods (Borzekowski, 2001). Preschoolers say foods with certain cartoon characters on the packaging are better tasting than the same foods packaged without the character depictions (Roberto, 2010). Food and beverage industries focus on consumer choice and personal responsibility as the cause of the nation's unhealthy diet. Health advocates argue that these companies also have a responsibility to provide consumers with attractive and affordable selections that contribute to the long-term public health.

Stakeholder Responses to Obesity Issues

A stakeholder is a person, group, or organization that has a direct or indirect stake or interest in a particular issue. The public health issue of controlling obesity depends on the collaboration of a broad range of stakeholders that could include:

- Private citizens
- Healthcare systems and the medical community
- Community organizations
- School systems
- Employers
- Health departments and health commissioners
- Local and national health advocates
- Local and national legislators and administrators
- Funding agencies (private and government)
- Educational and research institutions
- Privately owned businesses and industries

In a 2005 paper, George Bray, a professor at the Pennington Biomedical Research Center of Louisiana State University, described three strategies that stakeholders could employ to deal with the obesity epidemic: education, modification of the food supply, and regulation (Bray, 2005). Education about good nutrition, physical activity, and body weight can help the public understand the basics of a healthful lifestyle. Dr. Bray does caution that it is unwise to rely solely on the educational strategies currently in place because they have not been successful at preventing obesity so far. Modification of components of the food environment (smaller portions and less energy-dense products) may have an impact on the food energy that is available and acceptable to consumers. Regulation by communities, states, and the federal government should be directed toward creating an environment where it is easier to make healthful choices. For example, regulations about nutrition facts labels provide consumers with point-of-purchase information to compare and evaluate products. Healthcare providers, schools, workplaces, and government can apply any or all of these three strategies, and the food industry working together to help individuals and families achieve the best possible health behaviors.

Healthcare Providers

Physicians and other healthcare providers are often the most trusted source of health and food information. Patients are more likely to lose weight when they are advised to do so by their primary care physician (Ryan, 2010). However, a significant number of physicians and nurses consider themselves insufficiently prepared to treat patients with obesity (Brown, 2007). Many practitioners acknowledge that they will need to obtain specialized equipment and supplies to accommodate extremely obese patients. What is more, healthcare providers are often doubtful about how successful patients can be in weight-loss efforts. That pessimism is based on experience and awareness about the results of well-controlled clinical trials in which the average weight-loss tends to be modest while the recidivism rate is extremely high (Anderson, 2008).

Both self-report and experimental research demonstrates that clinicians often hold negative attitudes toward overweight or obese patients (Foster, 2003). Negative stereotypes about obese patients by a variety of healthcare providers include views that obese patients are lazy, dishonest, annoying, and noncompliant with treatment (Puhl, 2010). In a survey of 500 family physicians in New Jersey almost 80% of the respondents reported that extremely obese patients frequently lacked discipline, and 52% felt patients lacked motivation to lose weight (Ferrante, 2009). Other research indicates that providers spend less time in appointments and provide less health education with obese patients compared with thinner ones. Obese patients report that they feel disrespected by providers, that their weight is blamed for all of their medical problems, and that they are reluctant to ask questions about their weight concerns. While provider bias may be a cause of substandard healthcare experiences for obese individuals, there are other barriers, such as lack of knowledge about obesity treatments, adequate time to spend with patients, and reimbursement for care related to obesity prevention and management (Puhl, 2010).

Though providers cite time as a key reason for not providing weight-loss counseling, lack of knowledge may be a bigger barrier. In a study regarding obesity care attitudes and competency, 44% of physicians said they did not feel qualified to treat obesity (Jay, 2009). This perception may be a byproduct of the lack of training in management and prevention of obesity provided by most medical schools. As a result, practitioners are not well equipped to give advice to their patients. Stronger nutritional knowledge and more training in counseling skills would allow providers to be more effective in bringing about lifestyle changes in their patients (Pi-Sunyer, 2003). In addition, to provide suitable, quality care for extremely obese patients, primary care physicians could be better informed about medications and bariatric surgery, specific examination techniques, and obtaining insurance coverage for obese persons (Ferrante, 2009).

Apart from physicians, other medical staff also asked for more knowledge and skills in counseling and appropriate dietary interventions (Hansson, 2011). In response to patients' frustration with conflicting nutrition information and advice, there is a need for evidence-based guidelines that are easy to use and effective. User-friendly clinical weight management tools that can be integrated appropriately into primary care are increasingly available. Examples are the California Medical Association Foundation's Obesity Provider Toolkit and the clinical tools from North Carolina's Eat Smart, Move More program. Websites for these tools can be found in the Resources section of this chapter.

Another reported barrier is that staff members believe that primary care is not an appropriate setting for obesity treatment and that it is not their responsibility, particularly if no other medical condition is present. They considered that their main task was to treat diseases, and overweight and obesity were not seen in this context (Hansson, 2011). Insurers do not want to pay for treatments that are not guaranteed to produce effective outcomes and at this time there are few effective obesity treatments (Pi-Sunyer, 2003). Insurance reimbursement for obesity treatment is often easier to obtain when the patient is labeled as having a related disease such as type 2 diabetes or hyperlipidemia.

Obesity management by healthcare providers has the potential of being much more effective than it currently is. Obesity should be recognized as an important issue at all levels of the healthcare system using a team-based approach that includes physicians, dietitians, exercise physiologists, behavior

therapists, and bariatric surgeons. Additional ways to enhance care would be to promote cooperation with other stakeholders, such as social welfare authorities and commercial weight-loss organizations. The quality of obesity management depends on educating current as well as future healthcare providers, by focusing on evidence-based treatments, and increasing providers' awareness of the possibility of their own negative views and attitudes about obesity.

Schools

Because children spend a good deal of their time in school, each school day provides opportunities for students to learn about and experience healthy behaviors such as regular physical activity and good nutrition. One of the key actions in *The Surgeon General's Vision for a Healthy and Fit Nation* is creating healthy school environments. The goals are outlined in this excerpt:

> To help students develop life-long healthy habits, schools should provide appealing healthy food options including fresh fruits and vegetables, whole grains, water and low-fat or non-fat beverages. School systems should also require daily physical education for students allowing 150 minutes per week for elementary schools and 225 minutes per week for secondary schools. (Benjamin, 2010)

> Critics say that food changes are necessary because school meal standards have allowed for too much fat, sugar, and refined carbohydrates, and do not actively encourage students to eat fruits and vegetables. Among the proposed changes for school meals are to serve fewer potatoes, corn, and other starches, and more green leafy vegetables (Levi, 2011).

The Healthy, Hunger-Free Kids Act of 2010 authorizes extra federal funding for school meals and child nutrition programs and increases access to healthy food for low-income children. Because a major objective is reducing childhood obesity, the law requires schools to adhere to new standards for school meals and all foods and beverages served or sold in schools at any time during the day. This includes vending machines, school stores, and snacks sold in the cafeteria. The act includes innovative aims that include helping communities establish farm-to-school networks, creating school gardens, ensuring that more local foods are used in the school meals, and expanding access to drinking water in schools, particularly during meal times. See the website listed in the Resources section for details about the Healthy, Hunger-Free Kids Act of 2010.

State and federal governments set guidelines for schools to be eligible for funding although school districts typically can decide what policies to follow or implement. On the positive side, many schools have previously taken steps to eliminate or restrict "competitive foods," or those products sold on school grounds that are not part of official school meals. Competitive foods are typically sodas, chips, candy, and other less-than-healthful products (Story, 2009). On the negative side, most states have laws requiring schools to provide a certain number of minutes of physical activity or recess during the school day. However, on the local level these requirements are often not enforced or the activities are inadequate (Levi, 2011). In recent years school systems have eliminated or severely cut physical education classes to focus on academic subjects. To understand why physical activity requirements are controversial, researchers surveyed more than 300 California school board members. The survey showed that over 90% of respondents believe that physical activity is important for student health. Yet more than half said they were not prepared to improve physical activity policies in their district because of tight budgets, limited time in the school day, and competing priorities (Cox, 2011).

Two examples of innovative school programs to combat obesity are the HealthCorps and farm-to-school programs. The goal of HealthCorps, a nonprofit program modeled in part on the Peace Corps, is to get high school students to exercise more and eat better. The project was started by cardiac surgeon and talk show host Dr. Mehmet Oz. Through after-school activities HealthCorps coordinators encourage teens, their teachers, and their families to become health activists. The program helps teens and their schools establish connections with public health departments, food banks, community foundations, service organizations, and businesses. In some communities HealthCorps members have helped to improve the nutritional value of products sold at corner stores and to repair parks and other recreation areas. More information about HealthCorps can be found at the website listed in the Resources section of this chapter.

Farm-to-school programs bring local fresh fruits and vegetables to school cafeterias. Farm visits, cooking demonstrations, and school gardens and composting sites are often part of the strategy. Studies show that these programs improve students' diets by increasing consumption of fruits and vegetables and result in students choosing overall healthier options for school lunches (Levi, 2011). In interviews about the opportunities and challenges of working with local farmers for school food procurement, school food-service professionals described three motivators for buying locally grown food for their cafeterias: (1) the students like it, (2) the price is right, and (3) we're helping our local farmers (Izumi, 2010).

Worksites

In the same way that children spend a large percentage of their day at school, men and women who are employed in the United States also spend a significant amount of time at a worksite. In the past healthcare professionals concerned with obesity focused on modifying eating habits and physical activity at home and during leisure time. Although leisure time physical activity levels vary according to sex, age, socioeconomic status, and geographic location, overall they have not significantly changed over the past decades (Talbot, 2003). A shift in programming to focus on activity during the workday is now necessary because an increasing number of jobs require almost no physical activity. Because worker productivity and medical costs are associated with worker health and well-being, employers are becoming more aware of the need to help promote health within the workplace. Worksite health promotion programs are often designed to address a broad range of objectives such as smoking cessation, stress management, or hypertension reduction. They may or may not include weight control as a primary objective (Anderson, 2009). Education, environmental modification, and policy and regulation strategies can be designed to make a wide variety of healthy choices easier for employees.

Examples of information and educational experiences at work include nutrition and weight management classes, health-related information provided on the company intranet, posters or pamphlets, and group activities such as health fairs and health risk appraisals. Modification of the environment may include enhancing access to healthy foods through alteration of food offered in cafeterias or vending machines. Employers can enhance opportunities for daily physical activity by providing onsite facilities for exercise, supplying showers, and offering subsidized gym memberships, secure bicycle storage, or incentives to use public transit. Some companies have even introduced standing workstations and treadmill-style desks (see **Figure 10.1**).

Policy strategies that could be effective are an increase in benefits or a decrease in health insurance costs or paid time allotted for breaks or meals at the worksite. Employers can implement wellness programs and create incentives for employees to participate. Modifying physical or policy structures is an efficient way to encourage healthful behaviors because it affects the entire workforce or population, rather than individual employees.

Obesity is thought to be an important driver of costs associated with absenteeism, sick leave, disability, injuries, and healthcare claims (Ostbye, 2007). Overweight and obesity are associated with higher costs; however, few studies have demonstrated that weight reduction programs achieve

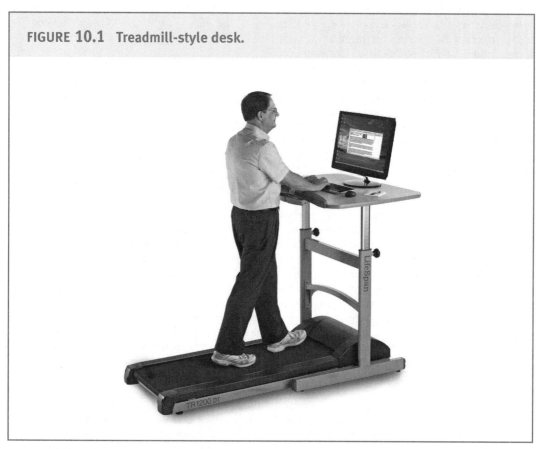

FIGURE 10.1 Treadmill-style desk.

Courtesy of: PCE Fitness - http://www.lifespanfitness.com.

significant cost savings in the short term (Blackburn, 2009). Furthermore, reviews have shown equivocal results on whether worksite programs for controlling workers' weight are effective. While evidence was found that worksite weight management programs confer modest, positive benefits, important questions remain. Which employee populations benefit the most from worksite health promotion interventions targeted at weight? Weight status varies considerably among employee populations. Most studies report weight or BMI change as group mean change. Therefore, it is not possible to determine if individuals at highest obesity levels benefited more or less. The question about whether a few employees lost a large amount of weight or if many employees lost small amounts cannot be answered either (Anderson, 2009).

To help employers determine whether health intervention programs will be useful for their business, the CDC has introduced LEAN *Works!* This is a set of online tools and information to help employers understand the economic consequences of obesity in the workplace and develop effective obesity prevention programs. A return on investment calculator is one of the tools to assess the costs and benefits of weight-loss programs. The Healthier Worksite Initiative website is another CDC product that provides interactive tools to help workforce health program planners design effective worksite obesity prevention and control programs. The Resources section in this chapter lists the website addresses for these programs.

Public Health

Public health professionals view the social, economic, and environmental conditions that promote and encourage behavior choices conducive to excess weight gain as modifiable factors. Public health interventions and policies such as educational programs to increase physical activity and regulation of advertising of foods or beverages to children are based on an understandable desire among politicians and health activists to reduce the problem of obesity, especially in childhood (Macdonald, 2011). Preventing obesity in children, and thereby reducing future risk of obesity in adulthood, is one of the most important public health issues facing the nation. Public health leadership

in innovative approaches and collaborations, partnerships, and coalitions at all levels, from the individual to the community and nation are needed to address this serious problem.

State and Community Government and Organizations

Because Americans live and work in public surroundings that have an effect on their health behaviors, responsible community policymakers and activists throughout the United States are engaged in creating healthier local environments. Availability of supermarkets and fresh produce, access to outdoor recreational facilities, infrastructures that support walking and bicycling, and safe neighborhoods are environmental elements that can be created or modified. Successful programs and policies to address these issues are those with flexibility to develop unique solutions to the health-related needs and challenges of residents in a given locale. Finding the means to develop and sustain such community improvements is a challenge. Clearly defined and sustained funding sources are a major hurdle for effective program implementation in most states and localities. Appropriate leadership, public awareness, and evidence-based research to drive policies are also necessary. For additional resources to implement neighborhood health interventions, states and communities often look to the federal government or private groups such as the Robert Wood Johnson Foundation, a philanthropic organization devoted to improving health and healthcare.

An example of federal government support for state and local action to improve nutrition and physical activity by changing policies and environments is the CDC Communities Putting Prevention to Work (CPPW) program. As part of the American Recovery and Reinvestment Act of 2009, the CDC provided $139 million to 50 states and $373 million to 30 communities and tribes to fund locally driven initiatives to help reverse the obesity epidemic. To see the list of funded communities, the wide variety of projects being carried out, and community success stories, visit the CPPW website listed in the Resources section of this chapter. Public health professionals have identified activities that are especially effective in modifying community environments. These evidence-based activities fall into five categories—Media, Access, Point-of-Purchase/Promotion, Price, and Social and Support Services. The strategies, known by the acronym MAPPS, provide an organizational framework to help communities promote health and prevent disease. Communities and states receiving CPPW funds must create a comprehensive plan to address healthy eating and active living through policy and environmental changes that involve the MAPPS

strategies. **Table 10.2** shows examples of goals for each MAPPS category.

The CDC has previously supported state programs through the Nutrition and Physical Activity Program to Prevent Obesity and Other Chronic Diseases (NPAO). The program works with partners across multiple settings such as childcare facilities, workplaces, schools, and communities to implement policy, system, and environmental strategies that have been proven to work for

TABLE 10.2 **Examples of Community Initiatives Based on MAPPS Strategies: Media, Access, Point-of-Purchase, Pricing, and Social Support.**

MAPPS	Nutrition examples	Physical activity examples
Media: Use media to increase awareness, knowledge, attitudes, beliefs, and social norms related to healthy behaviors.	Promote healthy food/drink choices. Limit advertising for sugar-sweetened beverages.	Promote use of public transit. Advertising to reduce screen time
Access: Increase opportunities for healthy choices and limit opportunities for unhealthy choices.	Reduce density of fast food establishments. Improve availability of food from farm to institutions, including schools, worksites, hospitals, and other community groups.	Enhance person and traffic safety in areas where persons are or could be physically active. Require daily physical activity in after-school/childcare settings.
Point-of-Purchase/ Promotion: Provide health information at points-of-decision.	Signage for healthy vs. less healthy items. Menu labeling.	Signage for neighborhood destinations in walkable and mixed-use areas. Signage for public transportation, bike lanes/boulevards.
Price: Leverage costs to incentivize healthy behaviors and discourage unhealthy behaviors.	Assess and balance relative prices of healthy vs. unhealthy items. Promote bulk purchase and/or competitive pricing for healthful foods.	Give incentives for active transit. Subsidize memberships to recreational facilities.
Social and Support Services: Provide services that facilitate healthy choices.	Encourage social support for replacing sweetened beverages with water at sports events and playgrounds.	Promote walking, hiking, biking in workplace, faith, park, and neighborhood activity groups.

Adapted from: MAPPS strategies CDC program Communities Putting Prevention to Work (CPPW) http://www.cdc.gov/chronicdisease/recovery/community.htm.

preventing and reducing obesity. The CDC Community Health Resources Database website has links to useful planning guides, evaluation frameworks, fact sheets, key reports, and state and local program contacts. To read about specific nutrition and physical activity interventions that states are developing or implementing, go to the CDC websites listed in the Resources section of this chapter.

Healthy Kids, Healthy Communities is a national program of the Robert Wood Johnson Foundation (RWJF) whose goal is to reverse the childhood obesity epidemic by 2015. The Foundation provides expertise and resources to organizations, policymakers and communities working to support affordable healthy eating and active living initiatives. *Healthy Kids, Healthy Communities* puts emphasis on reaching children who are at highest risk for obesity on the basis of ethnicity, income, and geographic location. Because RWJF's strategy for reversing the childhood obesity epidemic hinges on changing policies and environments, the foundation does not generally support projects that provide only information or education. Abundant information about RWJF policy priorities, its various programs, regions served, grant amounts, and directions for applying for funds can be found on the foundation's website.

In cities and counties policymakers have begun to recognize that access to healthy food is essential to healthy neighborhoods and healthy residents. Public policy interventions such as zoning modifications and grants or loans may offer supermarkets and farmers' markets incentives to set up their businesses in low-income areas and to offer affordable and nutritious food in underserved areas. For example, New York City implemented the Healthy Bodegas program in which bodegas, or small corner stores, in nutritionally vulnerable areas were recruited to increase their offerings of healthy foods such as low-fat milk, fruit, and vegetables. The city provided promotional and educational materials to entice people to purchase the new offerings and to encourage bodegas to participate (Ver Ploeg, 2009).

There is some evidence to support the benefits of renovating and restocking corner stores. Through the Healthy Bodegas program, 21% of the participating stores began selling low-fat milk and 45% of those reported that low-fat milk sales increased.

Further, nearly half of participating bodegas expanded their fruit and vegetable selections. A third of those stores reported increased fruit sales, and 26% reported increased vegetable sales (HBI, 2010). Comparable results were seen from similar programs in Maryland, North Carolina, California, and Apache reservations in Arizona. In the Apache Healthy Stores program, households located close to the stores that had the program were compared to households in outlying Apache communities. Customers who had increased access purchased and ate more of the healthier foods than customers who lived farther away. They were also more likely to decrease consumption of less healthy snacks and fast foods and sweetened beverages (Ver Ploeg, 2009). These studies provide evidence that store-based interventions can be an effective way to reach people in low-income communities.

Taxes

Perhaps the most controversial public policy proposition is to tax foods seen as promoting obesity. A frequently considered proposal would introduce a tax on sugar-sweetened beverages (SSBs), with all or part of the revenue designated for obesity prevention programs or subsidies for healthy food such as fruit or vegetables (Brownell, 2009). Because SSBs have become widely accessible, affordable, and available in stores, restaurants, and vending machines, this presents a realistic opportunity to use taxes to induce people to make healthier choices (Popkin, 2010). Thirty-four states and Washington, DC, have regular sales taxes on soda. New York, Philadelphia, California, and Massachusetts have considered implementing or increasing the existing tax on sugar-sweetened beverages. A suggested levy would be a penny-per-ounce tax on all nondiet soft drinks, including fruit drinks containing less than 70% fruit juice.

The health effect of taxes on soda and other SSBs is debatable. Many studies suggest that when these drinks cost more, people buy them less. A 10% increase in price leads to an 8% drop in consumption (Andreyeva, 2010). But few studies have found a connection between SSB taxes and weight loss. Another challenge for food taxes is defining the scope of what should be taxed. Should apple juice be taxed because it is energy-dense, or should it be subsidized because it is 100% fruit and sometimes contains added vitamins (Cawley, 2010)? In addition, community activists and the food and beverage industry point out that food taxes can be regressive, falling more heavily on the poor.

Liability Legislation

Another controversial issue is proposed liability laws that would prevent people from suing restaurants, manufacturers, and marketers for contributing to weight-related health problems. Corporations that were concerned about potential obesity-related lawsuits similar to the charges tobacco companies have faced have prompted the legislation. They want protection against claims that ask for compensation for individual health problems and also against those that aim to force the food industry to take responsibility for the health of its customers and to improve the nutritional value of its products. Members of the United States Congress have deliberated about whether the food industry should be protected from liability and frivolous lawsuits, and they have proposed bills limiting legal responsibility for causing obesity. In 2005, the Personal Responsibility in Food Consumption Act, known as the "cheeseburger bill," actually passed the House but did not receive a Senate vote and did not become a federal law (H.R. 554, 2005). Similar bills did pass in 24 states. Arizona, Colorado, Florida, Georgia, Idaho, Illinois, Indiana, Louisiana, Kansas, Kentucky, Maine, Michigan, Missouri, New Hampshire, North Dakota, Ohio, Oregon, South Dakota, Texas, Tennessee, Utah, Washington, Wisconsin, and Wyoming all have obesity liability or "commonsense consumption" laws. They vary somewhat in substance, but all prevent lawsuits seeking personal injury damages related to obesity from ever being tried in their courts (Levi, 2011). Proponents of these laws argue that obesity prevention is a matter of common sense and personal responsibility. Opponents argue that, in some cases, restaurants, food manufacturers, and marketers withhold crucial information about the adverse effects of their products and that industry profitability is more important than consumer health.

National Programs

The policies that were successful in reducing tobacco use in the United States demonstrated that comprehensive top-down strategies enhance individual education and treatment. Prior to 2008 the national approach to obesity was based on developing personal responsibility and educating about improved health habits and the dangers of obesity. After 2008 the federal government initiated a number of new or revised federal programs and policies designed to reduce obesity that addressed individual behaviors, as well as environments such as schools, worksites, healthcare organizations, and communities.

The Surgeon General's Vision for a Healthy and Fit Nation

In the 2001 *Surgeon General's Call to Action to Prevent and Decrease Overweight and Obesity*, former Surgeon General David Satcher warned of the negative effects of the increasing weight of United States citizens and outlined a public health response to reverse the trend. In 2010 Surgeon General Regina M. Benjamin said, "I plan to strengthen and expand this blueprint for action created by my predecessor. Although we have made some strides since 2001, the prevalence of obesity, obesity-related diseases, and premature death remains too high" (Benjamin, 2010). Comprehensive actions with more focus on environmental changes outlined in *The Surgeon General's Vision for a Healthy and Fit Nation 2010* include:

- Promoting individual healthy choices and healthy home environments.
- Creating healthy child care settings.
- Creating healthy schools.
- Creating healthy work sites.
- Mobilizing the medical community.
- Improving our communities.

An overall view of actions and suggested programs for each can be seen on the surgeon general website, which is listed in the Resources section of this chapter.

Let's Move!

Because coordination is essential among government agencies and other sectors in society, leadership at the national level is necessary to move a multilevel agenda forward. First Lady Michelle Obama assumed that leadership in 2010 when she launched the Let's Move! program, which had the ambitious goal of eliminating childhood obesity within a generation. The first lady was able to raise public awareness about the environmental aspects of obesity as the initiative brought together public officials, the food industry, advocacy groups, and others to find solutions. The Let's Move! website is a comprehensive resource for offers, tips, and tools for how to raise healthy kids at home and in schools. Accounts of the accomplishments that are occurring in cities and localities are updated frequently. The website is listed in the Resources section of this chapter.

As part of this effort President Barack Obama established the Task Force on Childhood Obesity to develop a coordinated strategy, identify key benchmarks, and outline a national action plan. The task force report presented a series of recommendations for addressing the problems of childhood obesity. The recommendations were structured around the same four goals of the first lady's Let's Move! initiative: (1) empowering parents and caregivers to make healthy choices for their families; (2) serving healthier food in schools; (3) ensuring access to healthy, affordable food; and (4) increasing physical activity (Let's Move!, 2010)

One of the task force recommendations addressed the issue of food marketing. It emphasized that "the marketing of food products can also be a powerful tool to drive the purchase of healthy products, and to communicate important information about healthy eating choices." The Federal Trade Commission (FTC) is charged with monitoring and evaluating marketing efforts that are meant to help reduce childhood obesity, and the task force report made it clear that the food and beverage industry should assist federal agencies, such as the FTC, in policing the marketing of food to children (White House, 2010). The report also includes several recommendations for the food industry, such as self-regulation policies to cover all forms of marketing, and limiting the licensing of popular cartoon characters only to food and beverage products that are healthy. While cartoon characters in advertisements and labels have been used to increase purchases of less-than-healthful foods and snacks, research shows that they can encourage children to choose fruits and vegetables. A study in collaboration with the Sesame Workshop showed that placing an "Elmo" sticker on broccoli led 50% of children in the sample to choose the broccoli instead of a chocolate bar for a snack. It must be said, and it is interesting, that nearly a quarter of the children chose the broccoli over the chocolate even when there was no sticker (Roberto, 2010). After the "Shrek" cartoon image was used to promote Vidalia onions, a trademarked sweet onion that is unique to southeastern Georgia, the demand for medium-size Vidalias, which typically fill Shrek bags, was up 35% (Jordan, 2010).

Affordable Care Act and Labeling

The year 2010 also brought the Affordable Care Act (ACA), which expanded benefits and coverage of services for obesity prevention and also had a section on nutrition labeling requirements. The ACA requires chain restaurants with 20 or more locations to post calorie and nutrition information on menus, menu boards, drive through displays, and certain vending machines. The Food and Drug Administration (FDA) was charged with making rules detailing how the law would be carried out. The benefit of readily available nutrition information on menus and menu boards is based on the consideration that informed consumers could make healthier choices. According to the Yale Rudd Center for Food Policy and Obesity, 80% of consumers want this information (Rudd Center, 2011). Leading health organizations, including the American Medical Association, also see the need for nutrient labeling that is easy to understand. Several states and localities led the way by enacting menu labeling laws before the ACA requirements were in effect.

It is not yet clear what effect such menu labeling has on food choices and obesity. Researchers examined the influence of required menu labeling on fast food choices in New York City where nearly 1,200 adults who ate at fast food restaurants were compared with a sample in Newark, New Jersey, which has no menu labeling law. More than a quarter of the New York City diners said the calorie information influenced their food choices. However, when researchers analyzed what diners actually bought, there was no difference in the number of calories purchased by the two groups (Elbel, 2009). In another study, researchers examined consumers' behavior at Starbucks coffee stores. The average number of calories per transaction fell by 6% when calories were posted prominently (Bollinger, 2010). Researchers found that in areas where menu labeling is mandatory, restaurants were 58% more likely to offer low-calorie options than restaurants in other areas.

Healthy People 2020

In 2010 the guidelines for *Healthy People 2020* were released. Healthy People reports are comprehensive documents of national health-related goals and objectives that have been published by the USDHHS every 10 years since 1980. The Healthy People goals are based on grades of scientific evidence. The Nutrition and Weight Status objectives for *Healthy People 2020* emphasize that new research should be directed to gaining a better understanding of how to prevent excess weight gain and to identify policy and environmental interventions that are most effective. Various programs may be popular and seem to show success, but the point is to find what programs really work if they are examined in a purely scientific manner. National leadership and government support can play an important role in facilitating and coordinating obesity research and supporting its translation into practical policies.

Strategic Plan for NIH Obesity Research

The National Institutes of Health (NIH) presented its second Strategic Plan for NIH Obesity Research in 2011. That version updated the first plan that was released in 2004. The new guide, which promotes a broad spectrum of obesity research, is framed around six overarching and integrated research areas:

- Discovering key processes that regulate body weight and influence behavior.
- Understanding the factors that contribute to obesity and the consequences of obesity.
- Designing and testing new approaches for achieving and maintaining a healthy weight.
- Evaluating promising strategies for obesity prevention and treatment in real-world settings and diverse populations.
- Using technology to advance obesity research and improve healthcare delivery.
- Facilitating the integration of research results into communities and clinical practice.

To increase the reach of research and improve public health, the plan emphasizes moving science efficiently from laboratory to clinical trials to everyday practice (NIH, 2011). Furthermore, research to identify and reduce health disparities is essential to all themes described in the strategic plan.

Many of these programs signal an understanding of the complexities surrounding the obesity epidemic and the need for collaborative efforts to successfully halt the progression of obesity or reverse current national trends. Multifaceted approaches that unite individual and community interventions with support from the public and private sectors are required.

Industry

As every segment of society plays an important part in reducing obesity the food industry and industries that shape the built environment should be recognized as essential partners. Specifically, this collaboration must affirm that these companies can respond to public and private concerns about nutrition and obesity while still meeting their business need to turn a profit (Huang, 2009). The Partnership for a Healthier America (PHA), an independent, nonpartisan organization, was created in 2010 with a mandate to mobilize the private sector, foundations, media, and local communities to action around the goals of the Let's Move! campaign. The PHA committed to bring healthy, affordable food to nearly 10 million people with new and expanded stores in low-income areas that lacked places to purchase affordable and nutritious foods close to home. First Lady Michelle Obama declared, "We can give people all the information and advice in the world about healthy eating and exercise, but if parents can't buy the food they need to prepare those meals because their only options for groceries are the gas station or the local minimart, then all that is just talk" (White House, 2011).

In the summer of 2011 Wal-Mart and McDonald's publicized plans to make major changes in the way they market their products and services: Wal-Mart announced that it intended to open 300 stores in areas without access to fresh produce and healthy foods, while McDonald's pledged to reformulate its Happy Meals. The new Happy Meal contained apple slices and 1.1 oz of fries instead of the original 2.4 oz of fries without any fruit. McDonald's had already made changes to its menu by adding new salads, oatmeal, and smaller portions of dessert in an effort to position itself as a healthier fast food chain.

In cooperation with the PHA the Healthy Weight Commitment Foundation (HWCF), a food industry–led organization, voluntarily pledged to change product offerings and make healthful foods more available (HWCF, 2010). The coalition includes hundreds of retailers, food and beverage manufacturers, restaurants, sporting goods companies, insurance companies, trade associations, nongovernmental organizations, and professional sports organizations. The members are held accountable and report annually to the PHA to ensure that their commitments are meaningful and sustainable actions to promote the health of the nation. The Robert Wood Johnson Foundation, a founding PHA member, funds a rigorous, independent evaluation and publicly reports its findings of the HWCF efforts to provide healthful foods to American consumers (Lavizzo-Mourey, 2009).

The Healthy Weight Commitment Foundation focuses on three areas: the marketplace, the workplace, and schools. Under its marketplace initiative, HWCF pledged to remove 1.5 trillion calories per year from the marketplace by the end of 2015. This reduction would bring the calories available in the marketplace to what they were in 2008. The foundation members pursued calorie reduction in several ways (HWCF, 2010):

- Product reformulation and innovation.
- Offering smaller portions.
- Redesigning packaging and labeling.
- Placing calorie information on the front of products.
- Providing consumers with information and educational materials.
- In-store promotion of the HWCF initiative.

The real challenge of creating new calorie-controlled products is that they must also satisfy consumer expectations for convenience, taste, quality, and price.

Summary

In an individualistic society such as the United States, making healthy choices is ultimately the responsibility of the individuals and families. However, the larger food culture and environment contributes greatly to the weight problems that are so prevalent in the population. The public health challenge is to acknowledge and build upon individual responsibility beliefs to generate personal and collective responsibility approaches in ways that will help reduce the incidence of overweight and obesity. It is important that local and national policy is shaped to help people make choices for a healthful lifestyle by removing obstacles and by creating more opportunities to be healthy. As Marlene Schwartz, deputy director for the Rudd Center for Food Policy & Obesity at Yale University asserts, "It's great for people to be responsible, but we have to make it easy for them. We have to create an environment that facilitates responsibility" (Hobson, 2009).

Researchers, experts, and government policymakers have suggested ways to change the food and activity environment to provide healthier options in communities, schools, and worksites. Many of these tactics are particularly aimed at underserved groups of people whose options have been most limited. Proponents of using taxes and laws to improve access to a healthful food and activity environment for everyone point to other government-directed public health successes. The theory is that if taxes and laws can get Americans to wear seat belts and to stop smoking, they can also persuade the general population to exercise more and eat better. The food industry and industries that shape the built environment are also responsible for creating an environment that will keep their customers healthy. Because consumers are becoming more interested in the benefits of nutritious foods and physical activity, creative and astute industry leaders can market and advertise attractive and healthful products that are part of a profitable business model.

New initiatives such as the *Surgeon General's Vision for a Healthy and Fit Nation 2010*, Let's Move!, the ACA, and other federal policy changes have provided new opportunities to support antiobesity efforts. Developing and initiating these programs is important, but that is only the first step. These policies must be fully implemented and funded. However, a tough economic climate creates new obstacles, particularly major cuts to federal, state, and local governments. As governments at all levels are facing difficult budget decisions, it is critical to think about both sides of the ledger: cuts to obesity programs today could mean higher health costs and a less healthy workforce later (Levi, 2011). The basic message from evaluations of previous and continuing programs and interventions is that reversing the obesity epidemic will be a long-term effort. It will require individuals, families, schools, communities, businesses, government, and other organizations to work together and to use new research to find effective ways to apply obesity-related science to practical, realistic applications.

Critical Thinking Questions

Question: What are pro and con arguments concerning the idea that obesity is an individual choice with individual consequences?

Question: What are some alternatives to the idea that parents of extremely obese children should face legal action?

Question: Consider the idea of taxing food that is thought to promote obesity. What are the problems and benefits that could occur?

Question: Is it surprising that McDonald's Happy Meals in France offer a choice of meat, fish, vegetables, mineral water, dairy products, and fruits? What are some reasons that the Happy Meals differ according to the country in which they are sold?(http://www.aboutmcdonalds.com/mcd/csr/about/nutrition_wellbeing.html)

Resources

California Medical Association Foundation's Obesity Provider Toolkit
http://www.thecmafoundation.org/projects/obesityproject.aspx
Eat Smart, Move More
http://www.eatsmartmovemorenc.com/
MyPlate Dietary Guidelines
http://www.choosemyplate.gov/index.html
Healthy, Hunger-Free Kids Act of 2010
http://www.govtrack.us/congress/bill.xpd?bill=s111-3307
HealthCorps
http://www.healthcorps.org/about-us
CDC LEAN *Works!*
http://www.cdc.gov/leanworks/
CDC Healthier Worksite Initiative
http://www.cdc.gov/nccdphp/dnpao/hwi/index.htm

Robert Wood Johnson Foundation Childhood Obesity Website
http://www.rwjf.org/childhoodobesity
CDC Communities Putting Prevention to Work
http://www.cdc.gov/CommunitiesPuttingPreventiontoWork/
CDC Nutrition and Physical Activity Program to Prevent Obesity and Other Chronic Diseases
http://www.cdc.gov/obesity/stateprograms/index.html
Robert Wood Johnson Foundation Healthy Kids, Healthy Communities
http://www.healthykidshealthycommunities.org/
Personal Responsibility in Food Consumption Act of 2005
http://www.govtrack.us/congress/bills/109/hr554
The Surgeon General's Call to Action to Prevent and Decrease Overweight and Obesity
http://www.surgeongeneral.gov/topics/obesity/
The Surgeon General's Vision for a Healthy and Fit Nation 2010
http://www.surgeongeneral.gov/library/obesityvision/obesityvision_factsheet.html
Let's Move!
http://www.letsmove.gov
Healthy People 2020
http://www.healthypeople.gov/2020/
Strategic Plan for NIH Obesity Research
http://www.obesityresearch.nih.gov/about/strategic-plan.aspx
The Partnership for a Healthier America (PHA)
http://www.ahealthieramerica.org/
Healthy Weight Commitment Foundation
http://www.healthyweightcommit.org
Rudd Center for Food Policy and Obesity
http://www.yaleruddcenter.org/
CDC Healthy Communities Tools for Community Action Community Health Resources
http://www.cdc.gov/healthycommunitiesprogram/tools/

References

Anderson LM, Quinn TA, Glanz K, et al. The effectiveness of worksite nutrition and physical activity interventions for controlling employee overweight and obesity: a systematic review. *Am J Prev Med*. Oct 2009;37(4):340–357.

Anderson P. Reducing overweight and obesity: closing the gap between primary care and public health. *Fam Pract*. Dec 2008;25 Suppl 1:i10–i16.

Andreyeva T, Long MW, Brownell KD. The impact of food prices on consumption: a systematic review of research on the price elasticity of demand for food. *Am J Public Health*. Feb 2010;100(2):216–222.

Barnett R. S.C. case looks on child obesity as child abuse. But is it? *USA TODAY*. July 20, 2009.

Barry CL, Brescoll VL, Brownell KD, Schlesinger M. Obesity metaphors: how beliefs about the causes of obesity affect support for public policy. *Milbank Q*. Mar 2009;87(1):7–47.

Benjamin R. *The Surgeon General's Vision for a Healthy and Fit Nation 2010*. Rockville, MD: Department of

Health and Human Services Office of the Surgeon General; 2010.

Blackburn GL. The ROI on weight loss at work. *Harv Bus Rev.* Dec 2009;87(12):30, 126.

Bollinger B, Leslie P, Sorenson A. Calorie posting in chain restaurants. National Bureau of Economic Research (NBER) Working Paper No. 15648, January 2010.

Borzekowski DL, Robinson TN. The 30-second effect: an experiment revealing the impact of television commercials on food preferences of preschoolers. *J Am Diet Assoc.* Jan 2001;101(1):42–46.

Bray GA, Champagne CM. Beyond energy balance: there is more to obesity than kilocalories. *J Am Diet Assoc.* May 2005;105(5 Suppl 1):S17–S23.

Briefel RR, Wilson A, Gleason PM. Consumption of low-nutrient, energy-dense foods and beverages at school, home, and other locations among school lunch participants and nonparticipants. *J Am Diet Assoc.* Feb 2009;109(2 Suppl):S79–S90.

Brown I, Stride C, Psarou A, Brewins L, Thompson J. Management of obesity in primary care: nurses' practices, beliefs and attitudes. *J Adv Nurs.* Aug 2007;59(4):329–341.

Brownell KD, Farley T, Willett WC, et al. The public health and economic benefits of taxing sugar-sweetened beverages. *N Engl J Med.* Oct 15 2009;361(16):1599–1605.

Brownell KD, Kersh R, Ludwig DS, et al. Personal responsibility and obesity: a constructive approach to a controversial issue. *Health Aff (Millwood).* Mar–Apr 2010;29(3):379–387.

Cawley J. The economics of childhood obesity. *Health Aff (Millwood).* Mar–Apr 2010;29(3):364–371.

CDC. Centers for Disease Control and Prevention. Basics About Childhood Obesity. 2010; http://www.cdc.gov/obesity/childhood/defining.html. Accessed July 15, 2011.

Church TS, Thomas DM, Tudor-Locke C, et al. Trends over 5 decades in U.S. occupation-related physical activity and their associations with obesity. *PLoS One.* 2011;6(5):e19657.

Cox L, Berends V, Sallis JF, et al. Engaging school governance leaders to influence physical activity policies. *J Phys Act Health.* Jan 2011;8 Suppl 1:S40–S48.

Dodd C. CAPTA Reauthorization Act 2010 (S. 3817). 2010; http://www.govtrack.us/congress/bill.xpd?bill=s111-3817. Accessed August 1, 2011.

Elbel B, Kersh R, Brescoll VL, Dixon LB. Calorie labeling and food choices: a first look at the effects on low-income people in New York City. *Health Aff (Millwood).* Nov–Dec 2009;28(6):w1110–w1121.

Ferrante JM, Piasecki AK, Ohman-Strickland PA, Crabtree BF. Family physicians' practices and attitudes regarding care of extremely obese patients. *Obesity (Silver Spring).* Sep 2009;17(9):1710–1716.

Foster GD, Wadden TA, Makris AP, et al. Primary care physicians' attitudes about obesity and its treatment. *Obes Res.* Oct 2003;11(10):1168–1177.

Hansson LM, Rasmussen F, Ahlstrom GI. General practitioners' and district nurses' conceptions of the encounter with obese patients in primary health care. *BMC Fam Pract.* 2011;12:7.

HBI. *Healthy Bodegas Initiative 2010 Report.* New York: Department of Health and Mental Hygiene; 2010.

Hobson K. If diets don't work, what's the solution to obesity in America? *US News & World Report.* March 5, 2009; http://health.usnews.com/health-news/managing-your-healthcare/diabetes/articles/2009/03/05/if-diets-dont-work-whats-the-solution-to-obesity-in-america. Accessed August 1, 2011.

Huang TT, Drewnosksi A, Kumanyika S, Glass TA. A systems-oriented multilevel framework for addressing obesity in the 21st century. *Prev Chronic Dis.* Jul 2009;6(3):A82.

HWCF. Fact Sheet Healthy Weight Commitment Foundation Initiative to Reduce Calories in the Marketplace. 2010; http://www.healthyweightcommit.org/news_media/media_resources/. Accessed August 15, 2011.

Izumi BT, Alaimo K, Hamm MW. Farm-to-school programs: perspectives of school food service professionals. *J Nutr Educ Behav.* Mar–Apr 2010;42(2):83–91.

Jay M, Kalet A, Ark T, et al. Physicians' attitudes about obesity and their associations with competency and specialty: a cross-sectional study. *BMC Health Serv Res.* 2009;9:106.

Jordan M, Schuker, L. The Onion's Best Friend Is an Ogre. *The Wall Street Journal.* June 28, 2010; http://online.wsj.com/article/SB10001424052748704123604575323433042544568.html. Accessed June 28, 2010.

Lavizzo-Mourey R. RWJF to Evaluate Efforts by Industry. 2009; http://www.rwjf.org/childhoodobesity/product.jsp?id=49349. Accessed August 15, 2011.

Let's Move! 2011; http://www.letsmove.gov. Accessed August 10, 2011.

Levi J, St. Laurent R, Segal LM, Kohn D. *F as in Fat 2011: How the Obesity Crisis Threatens America's Future.*: Washington, DC: Trust for America's Health; 2011.

Macdonald IA, Atkinson R. Public health initiatives in obesity prevention: the need for evidence-based policy. *Int J Obes (Lond)*. Apr 2011;35(4):463.

Malone K. Parents indicted on charges of child cruelty. *Marietta Daily Journal*. June 10, 2011.

McDonald NC. Active transportation to school: trends among U.S. schoolchildren, 1969–2001. *Am J Prev Med*. Jun 2007;32(6):509–516.

Murtagh L, Ludwig DS. State intervention in life-threatening childhood obesity. *JAMA*. Jul 13 2011;306(2):206–207.

NIH. NIH Obesity Research. 2011; http://www.obesityresearch.nih.gov/about/about.aspx. Accessed August 1, 2011.

Ostbye T, Dement JM, Krause KM. Obesity and workers' compensation: results from the Duke Health and Safety Surveillance System. *Arch Intern Med*. Apr 23 2007;167(8):766–773.

Papas MA, Alberg AJ, Ewing R, Helzlsouer KJ, Gary TL, Klassen AC. The built environment and obesity. *Epidemiol Rev*. 2007;29:129–143.

Pi-Sunyer X. A clinical view of the obesity problem. *Science*. Feb 7 2003;299(5608):859–860.

Popkin BM. Patterns of beverage use across the lifecycle. *Physiol Behav*. Apr 26 2010;100(1):4–9.

Puhl RM, Heuer CA. The stigma of obesity: a review and update. *Obesity (Silver Spring)*. May 2009;17(5):941–964.

Puhl RM, Heuer CA. Obesity stigma: important considerations for public health. *Am J Public Health*. Jun 2010;100(6):1019–1028.

Roberto CA, Baik J, Harris JL, Brownell KD. Influence of licensed characters on children's taste and snack preferences. *Pediatrics*. Jul 2010;126(1):88–93.

Rudd Center. History of Menu Labeling Laws. Rudd Center for Food Policy & Obesity. 2011; http://yaleruddcenter.org/what_we_do.aspx?id=124. Accessed August 1, 2011.

Ryan DH, Johnson WD, Myers VH, et al. Nonsurgical weight loss for extreme obesity in primary care settings: results of the Louisiana Obese Subjects Study. *Arch Intern Med*. Jan 25 2010;170(2):146–154.

Scaglioni S, Salvioni M, Galimberti C. Influence of parental attitudes in the development of children eating behaviour. *Br J Nutr*. Feb 2008;99 Suppl 1:S22–S25.

Schulte PA, Wagner GR, Ostry A, et al. Work, obesity, and occupational safety and health. *Am J Public Health*. Mar 2007;97(3):428–436.

Story M, Nanney MS, Schwartz MB. Schools and obesity prevention: creating school environments and policies to promote healthy eating and physical activity. *Milbank Q*. Mar 2009;87(1):71–100.

Talbot LA, Fleg JL, Metter EJ. Secular trends in leisure-time physical activity in men and women across four decades. *Prev Med*. Jul 2003;37(1):52–60.

Treuhaft S, Karpyn A. The grocery gap: who has access to healthy food and why it matters. PolicyLink & The Food Trust. 2010; http://www.policylink.org/atf/cf/%7B97C6D565-BB43-406D-A6D5-ECA3BBF35AF0%7D/FINALGroceryGap.pdf. Accessed July 25, 2010.

Ver Ploeg M, Breneman V, Farrigan T, et al. *Access to Affordable and Nutritious Food—Measuring and Understanding Food Deserts and Their Consequences: Report to Congress*. Washington, DC; 2009. USDA Administrative Publication No. (AP-036).

The White House. First Lady Michelle Obama Announces Nationwide Commitments to Provide Millions of People Access to Healthy, Affordable Food in Underserved Communities (Press Release). 2011; http://www.whitehouse.gov/the-press-office/2011/07/20/first-lady-michelle-obama-announces-nationwide-commitments-provide-milli. Accessed July 20, 2011.

The White House. White House Task Force on Childhood Obesity Report to the President. 2010; http://www.letsmove.gov/white-house-task-force-childhood-obesity-report-president. Accessed July 20, 2011.

CHAPTER 11

New Insights and Future Directions in Obesity Research

READER OBJECTIVES

- Explain why it is important to explore previously unacknowledged environmental factors that may have an impact on energy balance
- Recognize the role that gut microbiota play in energy harvesting and host metabolic homeostasis
- Describe how research in animals has led to the concept that specific viral infections may increase risk for obesity in humans
- Discuss the proposal that endocrine disrupting environmental chemicals may affect human fat metabolism
- Explain how sleep duration may be related to obesity and assess the validity of current studies of that association
- Provide pros and cons about the idea that obesity is socially contagious and list some social influences that could have an impact on energy balance in adults and children

CHAPTER OUTLINE

New Insights for Future Obesity Research

Obesity is a condition of disturbed energy balance. However, the energy balance concept does not explain why there is a drive to consume more than needed. Or, how is it that certain individuals are very efficient at absorbing and storing energy while others in the same environment do not gain weight? While diet and exercise are key factors in promoting obesity, it is clear that a variety of environmental aspects also play an important role in the process. To advance knowledge of potential agents involved in the development of obesity, investigators have studied the possible effects of such novel environmental factors as gut bacteria, chemicals and viruses, sleep patterns, and social relationships. The objective of these studies is not to discount or neglect the importance of diet and physical activity in promoting healthy body weight. Rather it is to help understand interactions between unacknowledged environmental factors that work together with an individual's genetic, physiologic, and behavioral makeup to affect energy balance. Following is a discussion of the role of gut microbiota, obesogens, viruses, insufficient sleep, and social networks in the development of obesity. **Figure 11.1** illustrates the associations among these factors.

Links Between Intestinal Bacteria and Obesity

SECTION OUTLINE

- *Introduction to Microbiota*
- *Variations in Microbiota*
- *Mechanisms of Action Related to Obesity*
- *New Discoveries Based on Microbial DNA Sequencing*

Microbiota Critical Thinking Questions
Microbiota Resources
Microbiota References

Introduction to Microbiota

Accumulating evidence suggests that bacteria in the intestinal tract play an important role in obesity and its related diseases. The gut is sterile at birth and is subsequently colonized with bacteria from the mother and the surroundings (Penders, 2006). Although the general composition of the gut microbial community is similar in all humans, there are specific variations influenced by age,

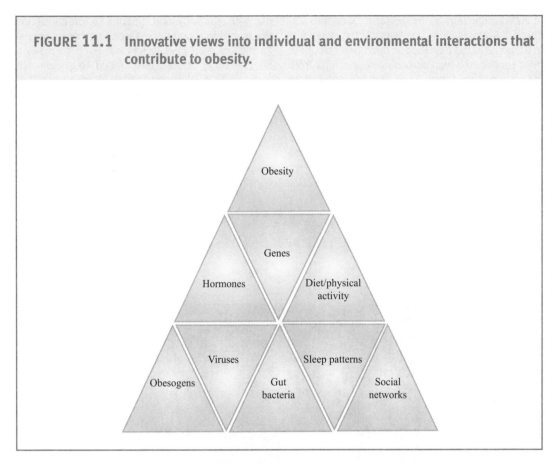

FIGURE 11.1 Innovative views into individual and environmental interactions that contribute to obesity.

dietary habits, and environmental factors so that no two people have exactly the same composition or ratios of bacterial species in their intestines. The trillions of microorganisms that normally exist in the gut vastly outnumber human cells. Although some of these microbes are pathogens, most are harmless and even beneficial. These organisms, collectively referred to as the **microbiota**, influence every aspect of human health as they perform critical functions that effect immunity, metabolism, and nutritional status (Sekirov, 2010).

The symbiotic relationship can result in a wide range of nutrient acquisition and energy homeostasis. As the gut microbiota harvests calories from dietary components that are not digested by the human or animal host, they obtain energy and nutrients for growth and proliferation. During the process they also supply extra calories for the host to use as energy or to store in adipose tissue for later use. Compared with lean individuals, those who are predisposed to obesity may have gut bacteria that are more efficient at energy harvesting (Cani, 2009). Scientists have found that germ-free mice that have been raised in a sterile environment and without gut microbiota had about 40% less body fat than mice with normal gut microbiota colonization even though the normal mice ate 30% less than the germ-free mice. The germ-free mice were protected against obesity (Backhed, 2004).

Variations in Microbiota

Another interesting discovery was that the ratios of intestinal bacteria in obese mice and people seemed to differ from that of their lean counterparts.

In 2005 researchers at the Center for Genome Sciences & Systems Biology at Washington University in St. Louis found that the gut microbiota of obese mice contained a high percentage of bacteria from the phylum Firmicutes. Their lean littermates had more bacteria from the phylum Bacteroidetes, the microbes shown in **Figure 11.2** (Ley, 2005).

The following year this group reported similar gut bacterial profiles in obese and lean humans. In addition, the microbiota of obese people who lost weight through a low-calorie diet shifted to resemble that of leaner people (Ley, 2006). Because many genetic and environmental factors can shape the microbiota array, the association of increased Firmicutes with obesity has not been consistent. Several other studies have failed to show such a correlation (Schwiertz, 2010; Jumpertz, 2011). Even though the altered Firmicutes/Bacteroidetes ratio may not be always linked with obesity, there is evidence that the gut microbiota of obese individuals contributes to increased fat stores.

Which came first—obesity or altered gut microbes? With a regard for ethical and practical considerations for testing whether the human

FIGURE **11.2** **Bacteroidetes are microbes that dominate in the intestines of lean mice.**

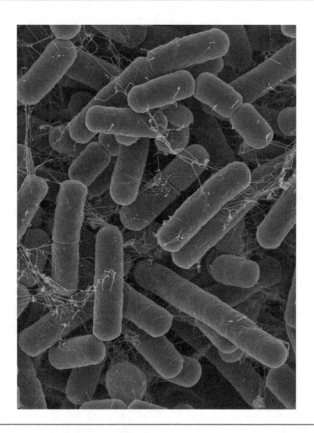

microbiome, or all the microbes in or on a human or animal, can affect obesity, scientists use germ-free mice as recipients of intestinal microbiota transplants from obese and lean humans to determine how energy extraction and fat storage may be altered (Backhed, 2011).To get insight into whether changes in the microbiota drive obesity or whether altered gut microbiota is simply a consequence of obesity, researchers transplanted fecal samples from the intestines of lean or obese mice to germ-free mice raised under sterile conditions and whose gut had not been colonized. After 2 weeks, animals that received the microbiota from obese mice gained a higher percentage of body fat and extracted more calories from their food than the mice receiving the gut microbiota from lean mouse donors. This work demonstrated that the tendency for obesity can be transplanted between organisms through fecal transplants and that the associations between the gut microbial ecology and obesity may be causal (Turnbaugh, 2006, 2008).

Mechanisms of Action Related to Obesity

To help elucidate why intestinal bacterial balance is a significant factor related to increasing fat stores, the microbiota of fat and lean mice was compared at the genetic level. Microbes from fat mice showed much stronger activation of genes that coded for glycoside hydrolases and polysaccharide lyases—enzymes that the human genome does not encode. These enzymes are necessary to extract calories from dietary carbohydrates (fibers) that would otherwise be indigestible (Backhed, 2007). Jumpertz and colleagues have assessed the relationship between particular gut bacterial communities and efficiency of food digestion and energy absorption in humans (Jumpertz, 2011). The group measured calories in food ingested and the energy lost in stools and urine in 12 lean and 9 obese individuals. A comparative 20% increase in Firmicutes was associated with about a 150-kcal increase in energy absorption, whereas a 20% increase in Bacteroidetes was associated with a decrease in absorption of 150 kcal. Apparently this variation in the microbiome has a small but significant impact on energy extraction.

The increase in the intestinal glucose availability and energy extraction from nondigestible food components may lead to higher blood glucose and insulin levels. These are two key metabolic factors that increase hepatic lipogenesis and promote adipose tissue storage. Animal studies of obese mice with enhanced capacity to harvest nutrients from a carbohydrate-rich diet showed that there was also increased production of another metabolic product: short-chain fatty acids (SCFAs). These can be used as substrates for lipogenesis as well as signaling molecules (Turnbaugh, 2006). The SCFAs or lipid metabolites are remarkable in that they are bioactive compounds that can interact with cellular targets to control immunity and energy metabolism. These signals produced by the microbiota circulate throughout the body and have wide-ranging effects. They influence nutrient homeostasis in the pancreas, muscle, liver, adipose tissue, and brain where they can influence satiety control in the hypothalamus (Reid, 2011).

New Discoveries Based on Microbial DNA Sequencing

Studies of gut microbe links to energy balance have introduced new ideas that may yield novel treatment strategies for obesity. As most current research findings in this field are based on mouse studies, their application to human energy balance requires further investigation. Scientists are beginning to think about differences in an individual's microbiota being analogous to human genetic differences. However, these microbial communities have been largely unstudied and their influence upon human nutrition is almost entirely unknown. Fortunately, technological advances have made the surveillance of human and animal microbiomes easier as it is not necessary to assess bacterial composition by culturing fecal samples. New techniques based on microbial DNA sequencing have allowed for huge numbers of microbes to be studied quickly and easily. As one of several international **metagenomics** analysis efforts to study genetic material from a mixed community of organisms, the National Institutes of Health launched the Human Microbiome Project in 2007 to determine what parts of the microbiota are similar in all humans and what parts differ—and how those differences may relate to diseases such as obesity. For more information about the Human Microbiome Project see the Resources section of this chapter. The next step to understanding the impact of the microbiota on health or disease is to go beyond the basic genomic inventories of the microbial species that live in the intestine to determine which proteins their genes express and the metabolites that eventually are absorbed. It is these functional end products that link gut bacteria and the impact they have on obesity.

Microbiota Critical Thinking Questions

Question: Discuss the pros and cons of transplanting bacteria from lean to obese individuals as a weight-loss treatment.

Question: Considering the obesity resistance of germ-free mice and the impact of the Firmicutes/Bacteroidetes ratio, what are some issues associated with human obesity and antibiotic use?

Question: How would you describe the possibility of gut microbial engineering, perhaps with particular exposures or foods that could be used as obesity therapy?

Microbiota Resources

Human Microbiome Project
https://commonfund.nih.gov/hmp/

Microbiota References

Backhed F, Ding H, Wang T, et al. The gut microbiota as an environmental factor that regulates fat storage. *Proc Natl Acad Sci USA*. Nov 2 2004;101(44):15718–15723.

Cani PD, Delzenne NM. The role of the gut microbiota in energy metabolism and metabolic disease. *Curr Pharm Des*. 2009;15(13):1546–1558.

Jumpertz R, Le DS, Turnbaugh PJ, et al. Energy-balance studies reveal associations between gut microbes, caloric load, and nutrient absorption in humans. *Am J Clin Nutr*. Jul 2011;94(1):58–65.

Ley RE, Backhed F, Turnbaugh P, Lozupone CA, Knight RD, Gordon JI. Obesity alters gut microbial ecology. *Proc Natl Acad Sci USA*. Aug 2 2005;102(31):11070–11075.

Ley RE, Turnbaugh PJ, Klein S, Gordon JI. Microbial ecology: human gut microbes associated with obesity. *Nature*. Dec 21 2006;444(7122):1022–1023.

Penders J, Thijs C, Vink C, et al. Factors influencing the composition of the intestinal microbiota in early infancy. *Pediatrics*. Aug 2006;118(2):511–521.

Reid G. The microbes are coming. *CMAJ*. Aug 9 2011; 183(11):1332.

Schwiertz A, Taras D, Schafer K, et al. Microbiota and SCFA in lean and overweight healthy subjects. *Obesity (Silver Spring)*. Jan 2010;18(1):190–195.

Sekirov I, Russell SL, Antunes LC, Finlay BB. Gut microbiota in health and disease. *Physiol Rev*. Jul 2010; 90(3):859–904.

Turnbaugh PJ, Backhed F, Fulton L, Gordon JI. Diet-induced obesity is linked to marked but reversible alterations in the mouse distal gut microbiome. *Cell Host Microbe*. Apr 17 2008;3(4):213–223.

Turnbaugh PJ, Ley RE, Mahowald MA, Magrini V, Mardis ER, Gordon JI. An obesity-associated gut microbiome with increased capacity for energy harvest. *Nature*. Dec 21 2006;444(7122):1027–1031.

Viruses Potentially Cause Obesity

BOX 11.1   Adenoviruses

Adenoviruses are one of a family of human DNA viruses that are most often associated with gastrointestinal infections, eye inflammation, and upper respiratory tract infections ranging from mild colds to serious pneumonia. The virus can be transmitted via air, water, or contact routes. Some infections with adenoviruses are promptly destroyed by the immune system whereas other types of adenoviruses are able to establish persistent asymptomatic infections in the tonsils, adenoids, and intestines. Shedding of the virus can occur for months or years after the initial infection.

Viruses and Obesity in Animals

Along with traditionally recognized genetic and behavioral factors, emerging evidence indicates that infection by viruses may be a potential cause of human obesity. Dr. Richard Atkinson, director of Obetech Obesity Research Center in Richmond, Virginia, writes about the obesity epidemic: "One potential explanation of the 'epidemic' is that truly it is an epidemic due to infectious causes, specifically virus-induced obesity, at least in part" (Atkinson, 2007). Dozens of investigations have shown a positive association between virus exposure and obesity in animals. In 1992 Dhurandhar and colleagues noted that SMAM-1, a highly infectious avian virus, caused development of an excessive amount of intra-abdominal fat in chickens without an increase in food intake. When the researchers inoculated uninfected chickens with the SMAM-1 virus, they found that, compared with controls, the exposed chickens had significantly greater body fat even though the two groups consumed identical portions of food.

Adenovirus-36

Further studies confirmed that adiposity could also be induced in chickens, mice, and monkeys by infecting them with AD36, a human **adenovirus** (Dhurandhar, 2000, 2002). In addition, the researchers reported that, along with the virus, obesity could be transmitted from infected animals to uninfected animals. Blood transfusion from obese AD36-infected chickens to nonobese, uninfected chickens resulted in subsequent obesity (Dhurandhar, 2001).

Viruses and Obesity in Humans

Although various microbes have been reported to cause obesity in experimental models (Pasarica, 2007), limited research exists to corroborate this association in humans. Considering the role that adipose tissue plays in increasing inflammatory response, a relationship between infections and obesity in humans is plausible. Adipocytes and macrophage immune function cells share many similar characteristics. They are so similar that, in some circumstances, **preadipocytes** can even differentiate to become macrophage cells (Charriere, 2003).

Demonstrating a cause-and-effect relationship in humans is complicated. It would be unethical to experimentally infect humans with these pathogens, so indirect methodologies have to be applied. For example, assessing the presence of AD36-specific antibodies in blood serum can test evidence of previous exposure to AD36. An assessment of humans using **serology** to determine previous exposure to AD36 was carried out at obesity centers in the United States. Scientists reported that 30% of obese (BMI > 29) and 11% of nonobese adults had AD36 antibodies (Atkinson, 2005). Similar to the adults, investigations in Korean children found a prevalence of AD36 antibodies in 29 to 30% of obese children (Atkinson, 2010; Na, 2010). A study in California also showed that AD36-positive children were more likely to be obese, and AD36-specific antibody status correlated with the severity of obesity (Gabbert, 2010). It may be that true causality exists between AD36 and obesity; however, Gabbert cautions that alternate explanations should be considered. Perhaps obese individuals are more vulnerable to AD36 infection because obesity itself is associated with immune dysfunction.

Not all reports have shown a positive relationship between AD36 exposure and obesity. There was no association of AD36 with obesity in a group of military personnel, although the researchers did find that the prevalence of antibodies was about 37% in 300 lean and obese participants (Broderick, 2010).

An alternative method of assessing the AD36-obesity relationship in humans was to look at how the virus interacts with human stem cells growing outside the body in laboratory cultures. Dr. Magdalena Pasarica at the Pennington Biomedical Research Center obtained fat stem cells from patients who had undergone liposuction and exposed the preadipocytes to AD36. As a result, the nascent fat cells differentiated into mature adipocytes with lipid accumulation. The ability of AD36 to stimulate **adipogenesis** in stem cells in vitro might indicate that a similar process could occur in vivo (Pasarica, 2008).

Areas for Future Research

At this time AD36 is the only virus that shows a potential link with human obesity (Atkinson, 2005). As not all individuals infected by AD36 become overweight or obese it is possible that genetic factors prevent or enhance AD36-induced obesity. Future genetic work could help to illuminate the mechanisms and the interactions between human genes, viruses, and energy balance. To convincingly describe AD36 as a significant factor in the widespread increase in obesity, it will be important to identify the underlying factors that connect obesity with this virus and eventually to find a way to treat it. If AD36 contributes to the occurrence of human obesity in any way, logical interventions would be to develop a vaccine to prevent infection or create treatments to reduce the effects after infection. Another area for further study is the temporal connection between the discovery of AD36 and the initiation of the worldwide epidemic of obesity (Atkinson, 2007). It may be useful to consider the virus hypothesis with respect to the time period in which obesity rates have increased and to determine whether AD36 infection rates do increase in parallel with obesity rates.

Viruses Critical Thinking Questions

Question: Discuss the social and medical consequences of the possible link between AD36 infection and obesity in animals and humans.

Question: Would you suggest that a person with obesity be tested for AD36? What would be the benefits and disadvantages?

Viruses Resources

Obetech
http://www.obesityvirus.com/
Obetech offers information and tests related to infection with AD36 in humans and animals.

Viruses References

Atkinson RL, Dhurandhar NV, Allison DB, et al. Human adenovirus-36 is associated with increased body weight and paradoxical reduction of serum lipids. *Int J Obes (Lond).* Mar 2005;29(3):281-286.

Atkinson RL. Viruses as an etiology of obesity. *Mayo Clin Proc.* Oct 2007;82(10):1192-1198.

Atkinson RL, Lee I, Shin HJ, He J. Human adenovirus-36 antibody status is associated with obesity in children. *Int J Pediatr Obes.* Apr 2010;5(2):157-160.

Broderick MP, Hansen CJ, Irvine M, et al. Adenovirus 36 seropositivity is strongly associated with race and gender, but not obesity, among US military personnel. *Int J Obes (Lond).* Feb 2010;34(2):302-308.

Charriere G, Cousin B, Arnaud E, et al. Preadipocyte conversion to macrophage. Evidence of plasticity. *J Biol Chem.* Mar 14 2003;278(11):9850-9855.

Dhurandhar NV, Israel BA, Kolesar JM, Mayhew GF, Cook ME, Atkinson RL. Increased adiposity in animals due to a human virus. *Int J Obes Relat Metab Disord.* Aug 2000;24(8):989-996.

Dhurandhar NV, Israel BA, Kolesar JM, Mayhew G, Cook ME, Atkinson RL. Transmissibility of adenovirus-induced adiposity in a chicken model. *Int J Obes Relat Metab Disord.* Jul 2001;25(7):990-996.

Dhurandhar NV, Kulkarni PR, Ajinkya SM, Sherikar AA, Atkinson RL. Association of adenovirus infection with human obesity. *Obes Res.* Sep 1997;5(5): 464-469.

Dhurandhar NV, Whigham LD, Abbott DH, et al. Human adenovirus Ad-36 promotes weight gain in male rhesus and marmoset monkeys. *J Nutr.* Oct 2002; 132(10):3155-3160.

Gabbert C, Donohue M, Arnold J, Schwimmer JB. Adenovirus 36 and obesity in children and adolescents. *Pediatrics.* Oct 2010;126(4):721-726.

Na HN, Hong YM, Kim J, Kim HK, Jo I, Nam JH. Association between human adenovirus-36 and lipid disorders in Korean schoolchildren. *Int J Obes (Lond).* Jan 2010;34(1):89-93.

Pasarica M, Dhurandhar NV. Infectobesity: obesity of infectious origin. *Adv Food Nutr Res.* 2007;52:61-102.

Pasarica M, Mashtalir N, McAllister EJ, et al. Adipogenic human adenovirus Ad-36 induces commitment, differentiation, and lipid accumulation in human adipose-derived stem cells. *Stem Cells.* Apr 2008; 26(4):969-978.

Environmental Obesogens

SECTION OUTLINE

- *Obesogen Exposure*
- *Endocrine Disrupting Chemicals Mechanisms of Action*
- *Embryonic and Perinatal Exposures*

Obesogens Critical Thinking Questions
Obesogens Resources
Obesogens References

Obesogen Exposure

In 2002 Paula Baillie-Hamilton, an expert on metabolism and environmental toxins at Stirling University in Scotland, proposed that environmental chemicals play a role in the development of obesity as she noted that the rise in obesity has paralleled the increased use of industrial chemicals over the last 50 years (Baillie-Hamilton, 2002). She contrasted how many of these products cause weight loss at high levels of exposure, although at low concentrations they can promote weight gain. In fact some of these compounds have been used in livestock production to fatten the animals. A growing number of researchers are exploring how human exposure to environmental chemicals may encourage increased body fat. Much of the work is based on the obesogen hypothesis with **obesogens** being described as chemicals that can disrupt normal developmental and homeostatic controls over adipogenesis and energy balance. Obesogens often act as **endocrine disruptors** or **exogenous** substances that act like hormones in the endocrine system, disrupting the physiological function of **endogenous** hormones such as estrogens, androgens, and thyroid, hypothalamic, and pituitary hormones (Grun, 2009). **Figure 11.3** shows the interaction between endocrine disrupters and hormones. Studies of endocrine disrupting chemicals (EDCs) have linked them to early puberty, impaired immune function, different types of cancer, and other diseases (Diamanti-Kandarakis, 2009). Because hormones influence metabolism, appetite, and the distribution, number, and size of fat cells, it is plausible that endocrine disrupters could have a significant relevance to obesity.

Some EDCs, such as phytoestrogens in foods, are found in nature, but industrially produced EDCs are believed to pose a more significant risk to human health. Common synthetic EDCs include bisphenol A (BPA), phthalates, and organotins. These compounds occur in a variety of products including plastics, food packaging, cosmetics, shampoos,

lubricants, pesticides, paints, and flame-retardants (Elobeid, 2008). Lipophilic environmental pollutants are resistant to metabolism and may be stored in body fats. People who work with pesticides, fungicides, and industrial chemicals are at particularly high risk for exposure and sequestration of EDCs. Because many of these substances do not decay easily, a chemical such as the pesticide DDT that was banned decades ago may remain in high levels in the environment. Furthermore, EDCs have been detected in environments far from the sites where they were produced, used, or discarded. The chemicals can be carried in water and air currents and via migratory animals to an otherwise uncontaminated region. A product such as BPA may not be as persistent, but it is so widespread in use that there is extensive human exposure (Diamanti-Kandarakis, 2009). BPA is used in plastic manufacturing so it is nearly ubiquitous in industrialized societies. BPA content is highest in clear, polycarbonate plastics, but it is also used to line cans, milk cartons, and other types of food packaging. It is possible for BPA to leach out of these containers to contaminate foods, beverages, and drinking water. Phthalate plasticizers and various perfluoroalkyl compounds (PFCs) are widely used as surfactants that stabilize mixtures of oil and water in hundreds of consumer products. Organotins are persistent organic pollutants that are widely used in plastics, as fungicides and pesticides on crops, as slimicides in industrial water systems, and as wood preservatives. **Table 11.1** shows examples of EDCs.

Endocrine Disrupting Chemicals Mechanisms of Action

The hormonal activity of these endocrine disruptors is thought to occur through a variety of mechanisms. The most commonly proposed mechanism is by direct binding to one or more cell nuclear receptors, such as the estrogen receptor. Work in several laboratories has established that phthalates and PFCs are **agonists**, or activators, for the peroxisome proliferators (PPARs) and retinoid X receptors (RXRs). These two nuclear receptors work together and, by binding to specific regions on the DNA of target genes, they act as metabolic sensors for lipophilic hormones, dietary fatty acids,

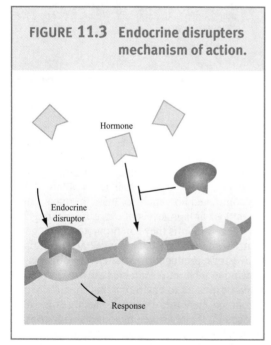

FIGURE 11.3 Endocrine disrupters mechanism of action.

Hormone

Endocrine disruptor

Response

Source: Endocrine Disruptor Research: It's Not Just Toxicology July 2009. http://www.niehs.nih.gov/news/newsletter/2009/july/extramural-update.cfm.

TABLE 11.1 Classes and Examples of Endocrine Disrupting Chemicals

Pesticides and fungicides
Methoxychlor
Dichlorodiphenyltrichloroethane (DDT)
Vinclozolin

Industrial chemicals
Polychlorinated biphenyls (PCBs)
Polybrominated biphenyls (PBBs)
Polybrominated diphenyls ethers (PBDEs)
Dioxins

Plastics and plasticizers
Plastics: bisphenol A (BPA)
Plasticizers: phthalates

Organotins
Dibutyltin (plastics)
Triphenyltin (agriculture)
Tributyltin (paints)

Natural EDCs
Naturally occuring chemicals found in human and animal food
Phytoestrogens, including genistein and coumestrol

Data from: Diamanti-Kandarakis E, Bourguignon JP, Giudice LC, et al. Endocrine-disrupting chemicals: an Endocrine Society scientific statement. *Endocr Rev.* Jun 2009;30(4): 293–342.

and their metabolites. Through this means they participate in regulating adipocyte number, size, and function (Grun, 2009).

Animal studies have supported the hypothesis that EDCs influence body fat accumulation. When pregnant mice were fed the organotins tributyltin and triphenyltin in doses equivalent to normal human exposure to those chemicals, their offspring developed more and larger fat cells than unexposed mice. Several papers in endocrinology journals have documented that alterations in adipose tissue development, lipid metabolism, and food intake are associated with phthalates, BPA, and other xenobiotics chemicals found in the environment (Grun, 2009; Somm, 2009).

Although evidence of the effects of EDCs on human obesity is limited, some epidemiological studies have found that chemical exposure is positively correlated with increased body weight whereas others found no consistent association (Lee, 2006; Nelson, 2010). Investigators who measured phthalate metabolites in the urine of adult males found that the concentrations were associated with abdominal obesity, increased body mass index, and higher waist circumference (Stahlhut, 2007; Hatch, 2008). It is apparent that further studies are necessary to sort out the discrepancies.

Embryonic and Perinatal Exposures

Due to wide environmental exposure, BPA has been detectable in blood of pregnant women and in amniotic fluid that surrounds the fetus (McAllister, 2009). Exposure to EDCs during critical periods of development can result in adverse health effects that may not be evident until much later in life. Embryonic development is in part directed by hormonal signals that control gene expression. An EDC-triggered abnormality of this prenatal programming may affect functions of organs and homeostatic systems for the entire lifespan. For example, **perinatal** modification of estrogen and testosterone signaling during fetal development can permanently impair reproductive system functions such as regulation of body fat accumulation. These early variations also have potential for transgenerational effects. Exposure during pregnancy can affect the mother, the fetus, and even the germ cells of the fetus, leading to alterations in metabolic and physiologic outcomes in the third generation and beyond (McAllister, 2009).

Although there is growing interest in studying the effects of environmental chemicals on human metabolism, currently only a few of the thousands of known environmental chemicals have been tested for their association with obesity. Furthermore, the vital cause-and-effect relationship between EDCs and obesity has not been demonstrated. To understand the role of these environmental obesogens there are numerous lines of investigation that should be followed to answer questions such as these (Grun, 2009):

- What are the adult outcomes of prenatal or childhood exposures?
- Can the endocrine effects on increasing fat cell size and number occur at any time in life?
- Are metabolic programming alterations permanent or can they be reversed?

Given that virtually all humans have been exposed to environmental chemicals and that so many questions remain unanswered about their influence on obesity, it is difficult to know what actions are necessary. Pediatrician Maida Galvez, who has monitored exposure to endocrine disruptors and body weight in a study of 330 children in East Harlem, says, "Even if these chemicals play a small role in obesity, it's a preventable exposure." She hopes that if environmental chemicals are shown to have deleterious effects, we can learn how to avoid them at critical stages of development and ultimately replace them with safer alternatives (Fraser, 2011).

Obesogens Critical Thinking Questions

Question: List some ways to reduce exposure to EDCs in your own food and lifestyle choices.
Question: Discuss the mechanisms by which environmental chemicals are intertwined with physiologic and behavioral factors associated with obesity.

Obesogens Resources

Bisphenol A (BPA) Information for Parents.
http://www.hhs.gov/safety/bpa/
Update on Bisphenol A for Use in Food Contact Applications: January 2010.
http://www.fda.gov/NewsEvents/PublicHealthFocus/ucm197739.htm
National Report on Human Exposure to Environmental Chemicals.
http://www.cdc.gov/exposurereport/index.html
Endocrine Disruptors.
http://www.niehs.nih.gov/health/topics/agents/endocrine/index.cfm

Obesogens References

Baillie-Hamilton PF. Chemical toxins: a hypothesis to explain the global obesity epidemic. *J Altern Complement Med*. Apr 2002;8(2):185–192.

Diamanti-Kandarakis E, Bourguignon JP, Giudice LC, et al. Endocrine-disrupting chemicals: an Endocrine Society scientific statement. *Endocr Rev*. Jun 2009;30(4):293–342.

Elobeid MA, Allison DB. Putative environmental-endocrine disruptors and obesity: a review. *Curr Opin Endocrinol Diabetes Obes*. Oct 2008;15(5): 403–408.

Fraser L. Is your shampoo making you fat? OnEarth. 2011; http://www.onearth.org/article/is-your-shampoo-making-you-fat. Accessed August 20, 2011.

Grun F, Blumberg B. Endocrine disrupters as obesogens. *Mol Cell Endocrinol.* May 25 2009;304(12):19–29.

Hatch EE, Nelson JW, Qureshi MM, et al. Association of urinary phthalate metabolite concentrations with body mass index and waist circumference: a cross-sectional study of NHANES data, 1999–2002. *Environ Health.* 2008;7:27.

Lee DH, Lee IK, Song K, et al. A strong dose-response relation between serum concentrations of persistent organic pollutants and diabetes: results from the National Health and Examination Survey 1999–2002. *Diabetes Care.* Jul 2006;29(7):1638–1644.

McAllister EJ, Dhurandhar NV, Keith SW, et al. Ten putative contributors to the obesity epidemic. *Crit Rev Food Sci Nutr.* Nov 2009;49(10):868–913.

Nelson JW, Hatch EE, Webster TF. Exposure to polyfluoroalkyl chemicals and cholesterol, body weight, and insulin resistance in the general U.S. population. *Environ Health Perspect.* Feb 2010;118(2):197–202.

Somm E, Schwitzgebel VM, Toulotte A, et al. Perinatal exposure to bisphenol a alters early adipogenesis in the rat. *Environ Health Perspect.* Oct 2009;117(10):1549–1555.

Stahlhut RW, van Wijngaarden E, Dye TD, Cook S, Swan SH. Concentrations of urinary phthalate metabolites are associated with increased waist circumference and insulin resistance in adult U.S. males. *Environ Health Perspect.* Jun 2007;115(6):876–882.

Sleep Disturbances and Energy Balance

SECTION OUTLINE

- *Changes in Sleep over Time*
- *Variations in Measurement of Sleep Duration*
- *Causes of Short Sleep*
- *Studies Relating Sleep Duration to Obesity*

Sleep Disturbance Critical Thinking Questions
Sleep Disturbance Resources
Sleep Disturbance References

Changes in Sleep over Time

Sleep duration may be an important regulator of metabolism and energy balance. Many experts believe that the number of sleep hours has decreased over the past decades in parallel with the growing epidemic of overweight and obesity. A study examining records of sleep and awake hours of full-time workers from 1975 to 2006 found a significant increase in the number of individuals who were sleeping less than 6 hours per night (Knutson, 2010). Polls conducted by the National Sleep Foundation (NSF) revealed that only 38% of American adults reported that they slept at least 8 hours per day in 2001. That number decreased to just 28% by 2009. In the NSF surveys individuals who slept less than 6 hours a night were more likely to be obese than those who slept 8 hours or more (NSF, 2009).

Not all studies support the idea that people are actually sleeping fewer hours and that short sleep and obesity are related. Horne and colleagues (2011) claim that the average number of hours of sleep has not changed much over the last 50 years.

BOX 11.2   How Much Sleep Do Adults Need?

Most research assumes that adults normally sleep for 7 to 8 hours a night. Although this is generally true, each individual has unique sleep requirements. Optimal duration of sleep need depends upon genetic, physiological, and environmental factors that vary across the lifespan. A basic definition of sufficient sleep is a sleep duration that is followed by a spontaneous awakening and leaves one feeling refreshed and alert (NSF, 2011).

This assertion is based on the fact that earlier measurements of sleep duration were not based on sleep time but on questions about whether participants felt "rested" and "energetic" when awake. Furthermore, Horne contends that the majority of obese people are as likely to be sleeping to excess as to be short sleepers (Horne, 2008).

Variations in Measurement of Sleep Duration

It would require large groups of people to be followed over long periods of time to explore the association between chronic sleep deprivation and eventual development of obesity. Long-term use of methods that are technically precise and accurate such as **polysomnography** or **actigraphy** is not feasible because they are also more costly. For this reason, large studies rely on sleep diaries and various questionnaires to collect data. However, self-reported responses about sleep are more likely to be subject to errors. In sleep data collection it is important to carefully define the multiple aspects that may affect how the duration of sleep is measured. For example, sleep habits can vary greatly between weekdays and weekends and large day-to-day variability in sleep duration may lead to substantial measurement error. The Institute of Preventive Medicine in Copenhagen has posed a number of pertinent questions about sleep duration and obesity (Nielsen, 2011):

- Is it duration of sleep as such or the resting time in bed?
- Is it sleep during the night or also brief sleeps during the day?
- Is it the regularity of sleep, the average, or cumulated duration over weeks or months?
- Is the match of the sleep with the biologic 24-hour or **circadian** rhythm important?

Causes of Short Sleep

Causes attributed to short sleeping are those associated with a lifestyle that includes frequent social activities, long working hours, shift work, and increased time commuting to and from work. Late-night television viewing and use of the Internet have also been associated with shorter sleep durations (Spiegel, 1999). As we live in a 24-hour society with wide use of artificial light, some experts believe that this exposure has the potential to disrupt natural circadian rhythms and adversely affect sleep (Magee, 2010). Many of these same environmental factors also lead to disruptions in sleep patterns in children. Physical and mental health status strongly predicts sleep duration. Medication use, pain, and mental health conditions such as stress and depression have been associated with reduced sleep (Magee, 2010). Obstructive sleep apnea (OSA) is a risk factor for both obesity and sleep disruption (Young, 2002). OSA treatments appear to improve sleep duration and additionally appear to be associated with significant reductions in visceral and subcutaneous fat after 6 months of treatment (Chin, 1999).

Studies Relating Sleep Duration to Obesity

A number of longitudinal studies have shown that short sleep predicts future weight gain (Gangwisch, 2005; Patel, 2006; Chaput, 2008). One of several investigations in which nurses in the United States were followed over a 16-year period found that those who slept about 5 to 6 hours a night gained significantly more weight than those who got 7 to 9 hours of sleep per night (Patel, 2006). In an intervention study in which sleep was restricted to 5.5 hours for 14 days in a sleep laboratory with free access to a variety of foods, participants increased calorie intake, snacking, and carbohydrate consumption. Most of the extra eating occurred in the evening and early morning hours (Nedeltcheva, 2009).

Exactly how short sleep interacts with weight gain is unknown, but two key hormones in appetite regulation, leptin, which suppresses appetite, and ghrelin, which stimulates appetite, are likely involved (Taheri, 2004). Young men who were sleep restricted to 4 hours in bed for two consecutive nights had significantly lower leptin and higher ghrelin levels compared to when they were allowed 10 hours in bed. In addition, their ratings of hunger and overall appetite were increased—particularly for high-carbohydrate foods (Spiegel, 2004). Leptin not only decreases appetite and increases energy expenditure but it is also affected by sleep time. Because leptin levels peak midway through a normal nighttime sleep period, sleep loss might contribute to lower leptin levels and increased appetite (McAllister, 2009).

Although short sleep duration is linked to weight gain, the association between chronic sleep restriction and obesity could be a case of reverse causation. Obesity may increase the risk of health conditions such as osteoarthritis, gastroesophageal reflux, and asthma that can disrupt sleep (Patel, 2008). In repeated sleep measurements of nearly 500 participants to determine if obesity contributed to chronic sleep restriction, weight was a better predictor of future sleep duration than sleep duration was of future weight (Hasler, 2004). Whether short sleep is a cause or just a correlate of obesity is not apparent. Further research from large prospective cohort studies with clearly defined and accurate measurement of sleep habits and repeated measures of both sleep duration and weight are necessary to demonstrate a causal link. To discover the pathways by which sleep curtailment impacts weight regulation physiologic studies in both human and animal models are needed (Patel, 2008).

Sleep Disturbance Critical Thinking Questions

Question: What kinds of responses from patients and clients would you expect from recommending longer sleep as a component in treatment of the obese patients?

Sleep Disturbance Resources

National Sleep Foundation
http://www.sleepfoundation.org/

Sleep Disturbance References

Chaput JP, Despres JP, Bouchard C, Tremblay A. The association between sleep duration and weight gain in adults: a 6-year prospective study from the Quebec Family Study. *Sleep.* Apr 2008;31(4):517–523.

Chin K, Shimizu K, Nakamura T, et al. Changes in intra-abdominal visceral fat and serum leptin levels in patients with obstructive sleep apnea syndrome following nasal continuous positive airway pressure therapy. *Circulation.* Aug 17 1999;100(7): 706–712.

Gangwisch JE, Malaspina D, Boden-Albala B, Heymsfield SB. Inadequate sleep as a risk factor for obesity: analyses of the NHANES I. *Sleep.* Oct 2005;28(10): 1289–1296.

Hasler G, Buysse DJ, Klaghofer R, et al. The association between short sleep duration and obesity in young adults: a 13-year prospective study. *Sleep.* Jun 15 2004;27(4):661–666.

Horne J. Short sleep is a questionable risk factor for obesity and related disorders: statistical versus clinical significance. *Biol Psychol.* Mar 2008;77(3):266–276.

Horne J. Obesity and short sleep: unlikely bedfellows? *Obes Rev.* May 2011;12(5):e84–e94.

Knutson KL, Van Cauter E, Rathouz PJ, DeLeire T, Lauderdale DS. Trends in the prevalence of short sleepers in the USA: 1975–2006. *Sleep.* Jan 2010;33(1):37–45.

Magee CA, Huang XF, Iverson DC, Caputi P. Examining the pathways linking chronic sleep restriction to obesity. *J Obes.* 2010.

McAllister EJ, Dhurandhar NV, Keith SW, et al. Ten putative contributors to the obesity epidemic. *Crit Rev Food Sci Nutr.* Nov 2009;49(10):868–913.

Nedeltcheva AV, Kilkus JM, Imperial J, Kasza K, Schoeller DA, Penev PD. Sleep curtailment is accompanied by increased intake of calories from snacks. *Am J Clin Nutr*. Jan 2009;89(1):126–133.

Nielsen LS, Danielsen KV, Sorensen TI. Short sleep duration as a possible cause of obesity: critical analysis of the epidemiological evidence. *Obes Rev*. Feb 2011;12(2):78–92.

NSF. National Sleep Foundation. 2009 Sleep in America™ Poll. 2009; http://www.sleepfoundation.org/article/sleep-america-polls/2009-health-and-safety. Accessed August 20, 2011.

Patel SR, Hu FB. Short sleep duration and weight gain: a systematic review. *Obesity (Silver Spring)*. Mar 2008; 16(3):643–653.

Patel SR, Malhotra A, White DP, Gottlieb DJ, Hu FB. Association between reduced sleep and weight gain in women. *Am J Epidemiol*. Nov 15 2006;164(10): 947–954.

Spiegel K, Leproult R, Van Cauter E. Impact of sleep debt on metabolic and endocrine function. *Lancet*. Oct 23 1999;354(9188):1435–1439.

Spiegel K, Tasali E, Penev P, Van Cauter E. Brief communication: sleep curtailment in healthy young men is associated with decreased leptin levels, elevated ghrelin levels, and increased hunger and appetite. *Ann Intern Med*. Dec 7 2004;141(11): 846–850.

Taheri S, Lin L, Austin D, Young T, Mignot E. Short sleep duration is associated with reduced leptin, elevated ghrelin, and increased body mass index. *PLoS Med*. Dec 2004;1(3):e62.

Young T, Peppard PE, Gottlieb DJ. Epidemiology of obstructive sleep apnea: a population health perspective. *Am J Respir Crit Care Med*. May 1 2002;165(9): 1217–1239.

Obesity Spreads Within Social Networks

SECTION OUTLINE

- *Framingham Heart Study Social Network*
- *Study Results*
- *Reasons for Social Influence on Obesity*

Social Networks Critical Thinking Questions
Social Networks References

Framingham Heart Study Social Network

A study published in 2007 in the *New England Journal of Medicine* reported that obesity looks as if it is socially contagious as it spread from person to person within a social network much like a virus. The study showed that when an individual gained weight, close friends tended to gain weight as well (Christakis, 2007). The research was based on a large network of individuals who had been part of the Framingham Heart Study. Weight, height, and other data were gathered from the records of more than 5,000 study participants at up to seven time points in the 32 years from 1971 until 2003. The research team had access to similar information from the records of the participants' parents, spouses, siblings, and children because most of the residents of Framingham were participating. In addition, in order for the researchers to be sure they did not lose track of their subjects, each was asked to name an unrelated friend who would know where they were at the time of their next exam. Altogether this group formed an intertwined social web totaling 12,067 people. The investigators knew who was friends with whom, as well as who was a spouse or sibling or neighbor. Because they knew how much each person weighed over three decades the investigators were able to examine an entire social network at once, looking at how a person's family and extended social contacts influence body weight.

Study Results

The results of the study showed that obesity spread within the social network and increases in an individual's weight correlated with weight gain in friends and family. People were most likely to become obese when a friend became obese. The weight of family members had less influence than that of friends, and there was no effect when a neighbor gained or lost weight. A close examination of the network showed that the obesity clustering was not just because people who were overweight sought to socialize with those of a similar weight. The investigators found that the likelihood of a person becoming obese depended on the nature of their relationships. The closer the social connection the greater was the influence on developing obesity. This effect of the social network extended, with progressively less impact, to three degrees of separation: to friends' friends' friends. Interestingly, proximity did not seem to matter. The influence of a friend persisted whether or not the friends lived in the same region. Increasing social distance decreased the effect, but increasing geographic distance did not. The same effect appeared to occur for weight loss, but most people were gaining, not losing, over the 32 years of the study. Consistent with the increase in obesity in the United States, the whole study network also grew heavier over time. A summary of the study findings includes (Christakis, 2007):

- Participant's chances of becoming obese increased by 57% if a close friend became obese.

- In same-sex friendships, a participant's chance of becoming obese increased by 71%. No similar association was found in opposite-sex friendships.
- Having a sibling becoming obese increased a participant's chance of becoming obese by 40%. This effect was more evident among same-sex siblings.
- Having a husband or wife become obese increased the likelihood of the other spouse becoming obese by 37%.
- Participants who were only one degree removed from each other socially, such as siblings or close friends, influenced one another twice as much as people who were two degrees removed from each other.

Reasons for Social Influence on Obesity

Analysis of study data suggested that influence on obesity status could not be attributed just to similarities in eating the same foods together or participating in the same physical activities. Not only did siblings and spouses have less influence than friends, but the remarkable impact of friends' weight seemed to be independent of proximity. "What appears to be happening is that a person becoming

---

FIGURE **11.4** **Eating as a social event.**

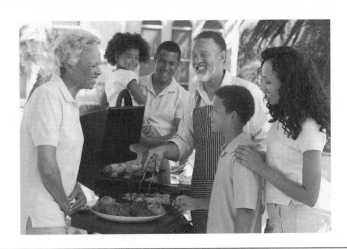

Source: © Hemera/Thinkstock.

obese most likely causes a change of norms about what counts as an appropriate body size," said study author Nicholas Christakis. "People come to think that it is okay to be bigger since those around them are bigger, and this sensibility spreads" (Obesity, 2007). This research, funded by the National Institutes of Health (NIH), was the first to provide a detailed picture of how social networks interact with other factors associated with the increase in obesity across the population. It did raise questions about *why* and *how* the network has such an effect.

Researchers at Arizona State University considered those questions by testing which social values shared by friends might influence perceptions of acceptable body size (Hruschka, 2011). Using data collected from 101 women and 812 of their social ties, the scientists confirmed Christakis and Fowler's finding that BMI and obesity did cluster by social networks. In contrast they found that shared social perceptions between friends play only a minor role in whether a person is obese. Though this survey did not look at extended relationships, their data suggested that other factors such as eating and exercising together may be more important in causing friends to gain or lose weight. They concluded that interventions targeted at changing ideas about appropriate body size might be less useful than those focusing directly on individual responses and opportunities for improving eating and exercise behaviors.

In another investigation of how social values may be related to obesity, a cohort of 288 young adult volunteers—described as normal weight (NW) with a BMI less than 25 and overweight (OW) with a BMI greater than 25—submitted questionnaires to determine weight, height, number of overweight social contacts, and their perceptions and opinions about obesity and obesity-related behaviors (Leahey, 2011). The data reinforced previous research in that obesity tended to cluster among social networks. Compared to normal-weight participants, those who were overweight or obese were more likely to:

- Have an overweight romantic partner (25% OW compared with 14% for the NW group).
- Have an overweight best friend (24% OW compared with 14% for the NW group).

With regard to the impact of the cluster viewpoint on weight and weight-related behaviors both groups reported low levels of social acceptability for being overweight, eating unhealthy foods, and being inactive. Among OW young adults, having more social contacts trying to lose weight was associated with greater intention to lose weight. These findings underscore that social connections influence acceptability of overweight and intentions for weight control in young adults.

Friendship may be especially influential in children and adolescents' eating behavior. A study of 31 boys and 41 girls between 9 and 15 years of age in Buffalo, New York, examined how overweight and nonoverweight youths modify food consumption depending on whether they are eating with a friend or unknown peer partner (Salvy, 2009). The authors maintain that youths are strongly influenced by their friends when determining acceptability of behaviors including eating. Their results indicate that both overweight and nonoverweight participants eating with a friend ate significantly more than participants eating with an unfamiliar peer. When eating together overweight friends consumed more than participants in all the other conditions. A conclusion about this experiment was that overweight participants might have decreased their food intake in front of unfamiliar peers to avoid embarrassment related to eating a large amount. Another inference was that the presence of an overweight eating partner might decrease an overweight youth's inhibition and result in greater food intake. Furthermore, individuals interacting with friends may have less need to monitor what and how much they eat to convey a good impression.

Regardless of the cause and effect, the intake of one partner influenced the intake of the other through some form of feedback loop or modeling factor. This work showed that youth use the amount of food eaten by their friends as an indication of appropriate eating. Repeated exposure to these patterns could shape common eating habits and contribute to similarity in weight status among friends. Whether deliberate or unintended health behaviors spread over a range of social ties. This interaction indicates that the social environment must also be considered when addressing obesity. It highlights the importance of treating obesity not only as a clinical problem but also as a public health issue.

Social Networks Critical Thinking Questions

Question: Describe an intervention for prevention or treatment of obesity that could take advantage of the observation that both harmful and healthful behavior might spread over a range of social ties.

Question: Discuss how a friend who lives nearby and a friend who is geographically distant affect your perception and values about obesity.

Social Networks References

Christakis NA, Fowler JH. The spread of obesity in a large social network over 32 years. *N Engl J Med*. Jul 26 2007;357(4):370–379.

Hruschka DJ, Brewis AA, Wutich A, Morin B. Shared norms and their explanation for the social clustering of obesity. *Am J Public Health*. Dec 2011;101 Suppl 1:S295-300.

Leahey TM, Larose JG, Fava JL, Wing RR. Social influences are associated with BMI and weight loss intentions in young adults. *Obesity (Silver Spring)*. Jun 2011; 19(6):1157–1162.

Obesity apparently affected by social networks. *Endocrine Today*. 2007; http://www.endocrinetoday.com/view.aspx?rid=24107. Accessed September 15, 2011.

Salvy SJ, Howard M, Read M, Mele E. The presence of friends increases food intake in youth. *Am J Clin Nutr*. Aug 2009;90(2):282–287.

GLOSSARY

Actigraphy: An instrument called an actigraph worn on the wrist or ankle measures body movement. It can detect patterns based on activity that are useful in assessing sleep-wake cycles.

Activities of daily living (ADLs): Daily self-care activities that require functional mobility, such as bathing, dressing, toileting, and meal preparation. Health professionals assess ability or inability to perform ADLs as a measurement of the functional status of a person, particularly in regard to disabilities.

Adenovirus: A type of human virus that commonly causes respiratory tract and eye infections; also may be associated with increased risk of obesity.

Adipocytes: Fat cells. Cells that primarily compose adipose tissue and specialize in storing energy as fat.

Adipogenesis: Formation of fat or fatty tissue.

Adipose (fat) tissue: Tissue that is stored underneath the skin as subcutaneous fat, intramuscular fat interspersed in skeletal muscle, and visceral adipose tissue deep in the body around vital organs. Essential fat cushions and insulates organs and is necessary for normal body function. Non-essential fat is excess energy stored away in fat cells for future use.

Aerobic exercise: Exercise that primarily uses the aerobic energy-producing systems; can improve the capacity and efficiency of these systems.

Agonists: An agonist binds to a receptor of a cell and triggers a response by the cell. It mimics the action of a naturally occurring substance.

Anorectics: Also known as an anorexigenic or an appetite suppressant, an anorectic is a medication or treatment that suppresses or causes loss of appetite and reduces food consumption.

Anthropometric: Refers to measurement of a person's physical dimensions—height, weight, and proportions.

Asthma: A common, potentially fatal, disorder in which chronic inflammation of the bronchial tubes (bronchi) makes them swell, narrowing the airways and causing breathlessness.

Bariatric: Pertaining to bariatrics, the field of medicine concerned with weight loss.

Basal metabolic rate (BMR) or basal energy expenditure (BEE): Energy expenditure for metabolism that accounts for 65 to 75% of daily energy expenditure and represents the minimum energy needed to maintain all physiological cell functions in the basal state. The principal determinant of BMR is lean body mass.

Behavior therapy: A form of psychological treatment based on the premise that emotional problems are learned responses to the environment, maladaptive behaviors can be unlearned, and new responses can be substituted for undesirable ones. Also called *behavioral therapy* or *behavior modification*.

Binge eating disorder: An eating disorder characterized by periods of uncontrolled, impulsive, or continuous eating beyond the point of feeling comfortably full.

Body composition: The term used to describe the different components that make up body weight. The components include water, lean tissues (muscle, bone, organs), and fat (adipose) tissue.

Body mass index (BMI): A calculation showing the relationship between weight and height that is associated with body fat and health risk. BMI = weight (kg)/height m^2

Built environment: It encompasses all buildings, spaces, and products that are created, or modified, by people. It includes land-use planning and policies that impact homes, schools, workplaces, parks/recreation areas, greenways, business areas, and transportation systems.

Cardiovascular disease (CVD): Any abnormal condition characterized by dysfunction of the heart and blood vessels. CVD includes atherosclerosis (especially coronary heart disease, which can lead to heart attacks), cerebrovascular disease (stroke), and hypertension (high blood pressure).

Childhood obesity: For children and adolescents (age 2–19 years), the BMI value is plotted on the CDC growth charts to determine the corresponding BMI-for-age percentile. Obesity is defined as a BMI at or above the 95th percentile for children of the same age and sex.

Childhood overweight: Overweight is defined as a BMI at or above the 85th percentile and below the 95th percentile on the CDC growth charts.

Chronic systemic inflammation: The result of release of pro-inflammatory cytokines and the chronic activation of the innate immune system. Low-grade chronic inflammation is characterized by increases in the systemic concentrations of cytokines such as TNF-alpha, IL-6, and CRP.

Circadian: Relating to biologic processes that occur regularly at about 24-hour intervals.

Cirrhosis: A chronic disease of the liver characterized by the replacement of healthy tissue with fibrous tissue and in which the liver is permanently damaged and scarred and no longer able to work properly.

Cognitive behavioral therapy (CBT): A therapy in which emphasis is on learning to recognize negative, irrational beliefs and then changing, or restructuring, thought processes to present a more accurate view of a situation.

Comorbidity: Two or more diseases or conditions existing together in an individual.

Computed tomography: A method of examining body cavities and organs by scanning them with X-rays and using a computer to construct a series of cross-sectional scans.

Cortico-limbic: Brain structures that are involved in cognitive, motivational, and emotional aspects of reward or pleasure.

Cytokine: A small protein released by cells that has a specific effect on the interactions and communications between cells.

Direct calorimetry: Measurement of the amount of heat (energy) produced by a subject enclosed within a metabolic chamber.

Edema: The swelling of soft tissues as a result of excess water accumulation. Edema is often more prominent in the lower legs and feet toward the end of the day as a result of pooling of fluid from the upright position maintained during the day.

Endocrine disruptors: Exogenous substances that act like hormones in the endocrine system, disrupting the physiological function of endogenous hormones such as estrogens, androgens, thyroid, hypothalamic and pituitary hormones.

Endogenous: Originating or produced within an organism, tissue, or cell.

Energy density: Energy density is the number of calories in food relative to its weight.

Exogenous: Derived from outside the body; originating externally.

Extreme or severe obesity (adults): A BMI greater than or equal to 40.
http://www.bcm.edu/cnrc/bodycomp/

Food deserts: According to the US Department of Agriculture, a food desert is an area where consumers are limited in their ability to access affordable nutritious food because they live far from a supermarket or large grocery store and do not have easy access to transportation.

Glycemic index (GI): An indicator of the ability of different types of foods that contain carbohydrate to raise the blood glucose levels. Foods containing carbohydrates that break down most quickly during digestion have the highest glycemic index.

Glycemic load: A ranking system for carbohydrate content in foods or meals based on their glycemic index (GI) multiplied by portion size.

Health at Every Size® (HAES): A health improvement and community-building program that focuses on self-acceptance, physical activity, and normalized eating without regard to body size.

Hedonic: Concerned with pleasure-seeking and related emotional or unconscious and autonomic drives.

High-density lipoproteins (HDL): Lipoproteins that carry cholesterol away from body cells and tissues to the liver for excretion from the body. HDL levels are inversely correlated with coronary heart disease risk.

Hirsutism: Abnormal growth of hair on a person's face and body, especially on a woman.

Homeostatic: Physiologic processes that allow an organism to maintain internal equilibrium and regulate bodily functions.

Ideal body weight (IBW): The weight that people are expected to weigh based on age, sex, and height.

Indirect calorimetry: A measure of energy expenditure as reflected by the resting energy expenditure (REE) by a subject by determination of the amount of oxygen consumed and the quantity of carbon dioxide exhaled.

Insulin resistance: The diminished ability of cells to respond to the action of insulin in transporting glucose from the bloodstream into muscle and other tissues.

Laparoscopic: Type of operation performed in the abdomen or pelvis through small incisions with the aid of a camera. It can either be used to inspect and diagnose a condition or to perform surgery.

Low-density lipoprotein (LDL): Lipoprotein that contains most of the cholesterol in the blood. LDL carries cholesterol to the tissues of the body, including the arteries. A high level of LDL increases the risk of heart disease.

Metabolic syndrome (MetS): A cluster of conditions—increased blood pressure, elevated insulin levels, excess body fat around the waist, or abnormal cholesterol levels—that occur together, increasing risk of heart disease, stroke, and type 2 diabetes.

Metagenomics: A rapidly evolving field that emerged from significant advances in DNA sequencing methods, with a focus on the use of culture-independent methods to study the structures, functions, and dynamic operations of microbial communities.

Microbiome: The aggregate genomes and genes found in the members of a microbiota.

Microbiota: A microbial community; commonly referred to according to the habitat that it occupies (e.g., the gut microbiota).

Mindfulness: Refers to being in touch with and aware of the present moment, as well as taking a nonevaluative and nonjudgmental approach to the experience.

Monoamine: A class of hormones or neurotransmitters such as dopamine, epinephrine, norepinephrine, serotonin, and melatonin, which have an amino group.

Morbidity: The incidence or prevalence of a disease.

Mortality: The relative frequency of deaths in a specific population; death rate.

Musculoskeletal: Having to do with the relationships and functions of bones, muscles, and cartilage such as those found within the hip, knee, and other joints.

Neurotransmitter: A chemical that is released from a nerve cell, which transmits an impulse from a nerve cell to another nerve, muscle, organ, or other tissue. A neurotransmitter is a messenger of neurologic information from one cell to another.

Obesogen: A chemical that that can disrupt normal developmental and homeostatic controls over adipogenesis and energy balance.

Obesogenic: Environmental factors that may promote obesity and encourage the expression of a genetic predisposition to gain weight.

Obstructive sleep apnea (OSA): A decrease in airflow when sleeping caused by a blockage of the airway, usually when the soft tissue in the rear of the throat collapses and closes during sleep.

Osteoarthritis (OA): The disorder, also known as degenerative joint disease (DJD), is a progressive degeneration of the joints caused by gradual loss of cartilage. The name *osteoarthritis* comes from three Greek words meaning bone, joint, and inflammation.

Perinatal: Pertaining to the period immediately before and after birth.

Perioperative: The period of time extending from the time of hospitalization for surgery through to the time of discharge from the hospital.

Pharmacotherapy: Treatment of disease through the use of drugs.

Polycystic ovary syndrome (PCOS): A condition in women characterized by irregular or no menstrual periods, acne, obesity, and excess hair growth.

Polysomnography: A test used to diagnose sleep disorders; also called a sleep study. The test records brain waves, the oxygen level in your blood, heart rate, and breathing rate, as well as eye and leg movements during sleep.

Postprandial: Following a meal.

Preadipocytes: Undifferentiated cells that can be stimulated to form adipocytes.

Resistance training: (May also be termed *strength training*, *muscle-strengthening activities*, or *muscular strength and endurance exercises*.) Includes activities that increase muscle strength by putting more strain on a muscle than it is normally accustomed to receiving. Often uses weights, weight machines, or resistance bands.

Resting metabolic rate (RMR) or resting energy expenditure (REE): The energy required to maintain all physiological processes while in a state of rest.

Satiety: The feeling of having had enough food or beverage; related to the length of time it takes before an individual becomes hungry again. This is in contrast to *satiation*, which means to satisfy or appease especially at the end of a meal.

Serology: The study of blood serum for evidence of infection by evaluating antigen-antibody reactions in vitro.

Serotonin: A monoamine neurotransmitter that plays a part in the regulation of appetite, mood, sleep, learning, and vasoconstriction. A low level of serotonin is associated with depression.

Steatohepatitis: A type of liver disease, characterized by fat accumulation and inflammation in the liver.

Steatosis: Accumulation of fat in an organ.

Stimulus control: Control of situations and other causes that trigger a problem behavior by methods such as avoiding high-risk cues, substituting stimuli that encourage beneficial behaviors, or restructuring the environment.

Stoma: An artificial opening made in surgical procedures.

Stroke: Sudden loss of function of part of the brain because of loss of blood flow. Stroke may be caused by a clot (thrombosis) or rupture (hemorrhage) of a blood vessel to the brain.

Subcutaneous fat: Adipose tissue lying directly under the skin layers.

Sympathomimetic: Describes a drug that mimics the effects of the sympathetic nervous system. It increases the availability of the neurotransmitter norepinephrine. This type of drug tends to reduce digestive secretions and appetite, speed up the heart, and contract the blood vessels.

Thermic effect of food (TEF): An increase in energy expenditure due to an increase in cellular activity associated with the digestion, absorption, and metabolism of food.

Thermogenesis: The production of body heat. Most body heat is a by-product of metabolism.

Visceral fat: Fat located in the abdominal area that surrounds the body's internal organs.

INDEX